The Language of Your Body

The Language of Your Body

Christina Valenzuela

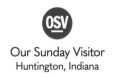

Our Sunday Visitor
Huntington, Indiana

Nihil Obstat
Msgr. Michael Heintz, Ph.D.
Censor Librorum

Imprimatur
✠ Kevin C. Rhoades
Bishop of Fort Wayne-South Bend
October 25, 2023

The *Nihil Obstat* and *Imprimatur* are official declarations that a book is free from doctrinal or moral error. It is not implied that those who have granted the *Nihil Obstat* and *Imprimatur* agree with the contents, opinions, or statements expressed.

Our Sunday Visitor, Inc.
200 Noll Plaza
Huntington, IN 46750
www.osv.com
1-800-348-2440
ISBN: 978-1-63966-051-3 (Inventory No. T2797)

1. RELIGION—Christianity—Catholic.
2. HEALTH & FITNESS—Women's Health.
3. RELIGION—Christian Living—Women's Interests.

eISBN: 978-1-63966-052-0
LCCN: 2023951835

Cover and interior design: Chelsea Alt
Cover art: AdobeStock
Interior art: Boston Cross Check, LLC, designua/123RTF.com

PRINTED IN THE UNITED STATES OF AMERICA

*The human body speaks a language
of which it is not the author.*
— Pope St. John Paul II,
Theology of the Body 104:7

+JMJD+
To my dear and loving husband, Andrés, and to our
children.
Colossians 3:14–17

Contents

Foreword

For many years, I subscribed to the notion that a menstrual cycle has no other purpose than pregnancy — so much so that, if having a baby isn't the woman's intention, she has the ability to completely eliminate her cycle without second thought. I also believed that hormonal contraceptives were the best and most convenient form of birth control. In medical school, natural methods for regulating fertility were only mentioned briefly but very clearly classified as unreliable. But this mentality changed drastically years later, when providential circumstances brought me to my knees and back to the Catholic Church.

Then I learned about a revolutionary medical field that challenged everything I knew about women's health. I was introduced to the concept of "fertility awareness," the foundation of evidence-based methods of family planning that can aid in diagnosing conditions that otherwise would have been masked by hormonal contraceptives. This new understanding made such an impact on me that my career was transformed into a ministry of helping women appreciate their bodies through cycle charting and the practice of Natural Family Planning (NFP). At that point, I had already earned my degree as a Doctor of Medicine, so it was quite the leap of faith I was taking. But as intrigued as I was about the science behind fertility awareness, I was drawn to a much deeper truth: our cycles not only tell the story of our bodies as a whole, but can also help us discover our worth and dignity as women. Moreover, a woman's cycle beholds a mystery that can draw her near to her creator. And this is precisely what Christina wants us to consider and embrace in this book.

Christina Valenzuela is one of the most dedicated, knowledgeable, and generous women I've had the pleasure to work with. We've collaborated on several different projects, including the translation of her course "Charting for Girls" (*Leyendo tu Ciclo para Chicas*). Christina has been a cycle educator for more than a decade and is a certified Boston Cross Check instructor. She has created several programs to help Catholic parishes with NFP formation, as well as to help parents and their daughters develop a positive attitude around their bodies and menstrual cycles. Christina has been very intentional in making sure her publications are accurate and reviewed by experts in different fields. But what sets her apart, and what I think gives her a unique perspective to write this book, is how her life reflects her Catholic faith lived through a Dominican spirituality.

Christina has gifted us with the book I wish I had fifteen years ago. It will make you ponder, wonder, and re-evaluate some claims that the world has sold women as "truth." Far too many have settled to live our womanhood in the shadows because we haven't dared to embrace the value of our menstrual cycles. Women have been cultured to see the menstrual cycle as an inconvenience, a stumbling block in the way of our dreams. But this book offers hope: our cycles are *good*. They are the window into our health, and they give us the ability to be co-creators of human life.

The Language of Your Body: Embracing God's Design for Your Cycle elevates this conversation so that we may begin to experience our cycles in a new way and understand how they reflect God's purpose of being in eternal relationship with us. I was thirty years old when I understood, for the very first time, that my cycles are more than a period, that my body speaks through my cycles, and that my fertility is a perfectly designed gift, not a burden. Had I known this much earlier in life, I would've saved myself a lot of heartache. I also learned that too many women share my story and come to this realization a decade too late. This is why I am incredibly honored to endorse the book you're about to read; it is truly a source of light and direction for women seeking to make sense of the complex but unique nature of their cycles and what it means to be a woman created in the image of God.

— Dr. Ross A. Bones-Castro, MD, MBA, FCP

Introduction

"My cycles are fairly regular and pretty easy. I've never had painful periods before."

"I suffered from agonizing pain for over ten years until my doctor diagnosed me with endometriosis. I have had three surgeries so far. The pain is better, but I'm worried about the potential impact on my fertility."

"For a while in college, I stopped having a period altogether because I was a student athlete. I didn't get my cycle back until after I graduated and started working, but my cycle is super irregular and I never know what's going on."

"I haven't had a period in years, thanks to pregnancy and nursing! I'm worried about what they will be like when they come back, but also kind of excited."

"I had to wean my baby early because my body just could not function without my cycle. I tried hormone supplementation, but the depression was so bad, I couldn't wait to get my cycle back!"

"I used to throw up every single month when I got my period.

The pain was so severe, I passed out a number of times. They put me on birth control, but it didn't help."

These are the real stories of women — snapshots of interviews and exchanges I have had over the past decade in my work as a Natural Family Planning instructor. Well, actually, the last quote is me.

It might be easy to assume that someone who writes a book about finding theological goodness in our menstrual cycles is someone who has easily found goodness in her own cycle, but the truth is that I have always struggled with the specifically female functions of my body. As a teenager, my periods were heavy and painfully debilitating, but I lacked the knowledge to express the level of suffering I experienced — and my doctors didn't have any suggestions other than artificial hormones, which didn't really help. I almost didn't meet my husband because I was laid up all that day, puking my guts out with cramps and a menstrual migraine.

I say these things not to write any sort of memoir or focus attention on my story over your own, but to assure you that I understand your objections to practically everything I am about to posit about the goodness and the beauty of our menstrual cycles. For many women — though certainly not for all — cycles are often experiences of pain, grief, and anger. To state the painfully obvious, they are also a bloody mess. It is easy to see how women and men may have come to the conclusion that periods could aptly be labeled the "woman's curse."

But there is something in our heart, soul, and mind that wants to be able to claim this bodily function for good. When I talk with other mothers about handing on cycle education to our daughters, the sentiment is almost unanimous that we don't want to fill their heads with fear, anxiety, or the sense of being doomed to suffering. We intuit that there is something strange, strong, and beautiful at work in our menstrual cycles — yet that positive inclination is often at odds with what we have experienced personally or seen among our female friends and family. In short, we experience a sort of chasm between how things *are* and how they *ought to be.*

For the Christian, this is the paradox and the tension of all life here on earth, the source of all suffering. Despite the fact that our bodies are created good, we experience bodily sickness, illness, pain, and death. Goodness can be obscured by these experiences, but it is not lost.

As Catholics, we have to start from the premise that God made everything good; but that in no way negates the fact that we live in a broken world … a world that we broke. Pope St. John Paul II wrote:

> Christianity proclaims the essential good of existence and the good of that which exists, acknowledges the goodness of the Creator and proclaims the good of creatures. Man suffers on account of evil, which is a certain lack, limitation, or distortion of good. We could say that man suffers because of a good in which he does not share, from which in a certain sense he is cut off, or of which he has deprived himself. He particularly suffers when he ought — in the normal order of things — to have a share in this good and does not have it.
>
> Thus, in the Christian view, the reality of suffering is explained through evil, which always, in some way, refers to a good. (*Salvifici Doloris*, 7)

While we may experience issues with our cycles that put us face-to-face with the reality that we are desperately in need of a Divine Physician, we still cling to the goodness. We have to ask ourselves: What good can we find in our cycles, specifically when we ponder the fact that both men and women are equally made in the image and likeness of God? It is this precise question I hope to unpack here, and to offer a few guideposts for your journey as you come to learn more about this unique aspect of God's design for your body.

We can also talk about a different type of suffering that is not directly physical. Even if our cycles themselves are healthy and well-functioning, we still live in a world that is primed to see our periods as somehow "unclean," which can mean they are a hindrance to fully participating in the spiritual life or, even worse, become a source of shame. Our own Church has sometimes directly contributed to these messages; however, as Christians who understand and appreciate the truths of science, it is right and just that we enter into a new consideration of cycles in light of information gained through the developments of medicine, biology, and anatomy. We have the opportunity to experience a sort of "unveiling" of the hidden work our body does, something that was not possible even a few decades ago! Specifically, we have the opportunity to speak meaningfully of menstrual cycles in their entirety, rather than just focusing on period bleeds. We have learned much in recent years about the often-invisible elements of the whole cycle, and this hiddenness — what we might call the *cyclical interiority* of the woman's body — is now ripe for exploration.

In the literature of our Church, there is very little that speaks directly about cycles. I have found myself wondering: If the male body experienced a significant biological event every month that utilized a huge amount of nutrient resources, created obstacles for exercising daily duties for about one out of every four or five weeks, and manifested as significant shifts in energy levels and moods, do you think our Church Fathers would have been silent about it? Would they have felt like they needed to hide this crucial part of their existence out of a sense of shame? Perhaps not.

What we *do* have in the Church is a rich theology of motherhood, both spiritual and biological, which is truly important. From the biological perspective of motherhood, we have gorgeous images of pregnant and nursing Mary to aid us in prayer as we contemplate how God is like a mother, and how God the Son desired to grow and be nourished by a human woman. On the spiritual side, we can talk about the self-gift of women who exhibit a special sort of concern for nurturing and cultivating goodness and holiness in the other. This type of spiritual motherhood is the calling of all women, regardless of whether they become biological mothers.

However, in the very strict sense, biological motherhood cannot happen without the key event in the menstrual cycle: ovulation. And the vast majority of spiritual mothers, even those who never conceive biological children, still experience menstrual cycles. It's not as if God, in receiving a woman's final profession into consecrated virginity or religious life, switches off her cycles. In touching the hem of her Divine Spouse's robe, her flow of blood is not dried up — because, unlike the woman in the Gospels who hemorrhaged for twelve years, her natural cycle is not a sickness. Religious sisters and nuns will live with their cycles in both the spiritual and biological dimensions until natural menopause, in the context of community life with other women who are experiencing the same.

So just as I want to be clear that we'll be talking about cycles rather than exclusively thinking about periods, I also want to be clear that we will not be focusing exclusively on pregnancy. Our understanding of motherhood in both its biological and spiritual dimension will be *enhanced* if we take time to understand cycles themselves — seriously thinking about the meaning of cycles when we have them as teens, as single women, as infertile women, and as women religious, and even when those cycles stop in menopause.

In order to dive into those questions together, we need to proceed in stages. First, we need to speak openly about the challenges we face as a Church when it comes to reverently exploring our bodies in a world that can be so hostile to seeing the body through that lens. I have encountered many Catholics of various backgrounds and opinions who aren't quite convinced that this is a topic the Church should spend time and energy on. So we'll lay a groundwork that first explains what menstrual cycles are and then put forward some important reasons why the Church *does* need to pray, think, and speak about this topic.

Next, we will need to recover a sense of the sacramentality of our bodies, by looking at how our cycles fit into the idea that both men and women were created in the image of God. We'll explore various lenses through which "cycles" can help us contemplate who God is, and who we — as humans, as women, and as individuals — were created to be.

And finally, we will explore what aspects of life might be different if girls and women were able to observe, chart, and interpret their cycles as a vital part of who we were made to be. What difference could this possibly make in my relationships? Does it matter in my friendships, marriage, or community life that I have this cyclical interiority? Can becoming literate about this particular bodily function actually help me grow in holiness? (Yes, it can!)

You may find that, depending on your personal situation or previous background with cycle knowledge, some of these sections may resonate with you more than others. You may find a richness in contemplating the "sign" of your cycle as a theological concept, but not really be interested in learning about the practical applications for charting. Or you may really be interested in charting and not care all that much about the theological reflection. Wherever you are in your relationship with your body and regardless of what knowledge you are particularly yearning for, you and your questions are very welcome here!

I also want to be careful to never suggest that "womanhood" is only (or even primarily!) expressed through our menstrual cycles. There are plenty of women who have had hysterectomies or who have already gone through menopause and no longer have cycles. Womanhood is much bigger than this single function. And yet, the ordering of the female body toward this potential to create and be a home for new life — even when that potential is not actualized — is a key part of understanding what makes women essentially different from men. Thus, my project here is not meant to exclude any woman who does not have a cycle, but rather to make sure that this element of woman's biology is not left out of our theological reflection on the way women image God.

No matter our vocational paths, for most of us — whether single, consecrated, or married — our menstrual cycles are present throughout a large part of our existence here on earth. It is a part of how God designed us as women, and therefore it is worth our time to contemplate what meaning is written into this aspect of womanhood.

Let us end this introduction, then, with a prayer:

In the name of the Father, and of the Son, and of the Holy Spirit.
> Holy Spirit, we ask that you come into our presence,
>> to hold for us any hurts, suffering, or negativity we have toward our bodies.
> Help us to see the goodness of our design as women,
>> to know deeply of the love our Father has for us as His beloved daughters.
> Open our hearts and minds to receive the truths hidden in the mystery of our womanhood,
>> that we may better know, love, and serve our Creator,
>> in whose divine image we are made.

We especially ask for the intercession of our Blessed Mother in this task,
and entrust these, and all things, to your Beloved Son, our Lord, Jesus Christ. Amen.

CHAPTER 1

What Are Cycles?

What are we talking about when we use the phrase *menstrual cycle*? It's not uncommon for a new client to come and explain to me that she regularly has six-day "cycles" or to explain that she is "on her cycle" right now. Of course, what she means is that her bleeds typically last for six days, or that she is currently experiencing her period bleed. But a period is only one part of a vast and intricate process called the menstrual cycle — the way a woman's reproductive system actively prepares for pregnancy.

To put it simply, the process of the menstrual cycle can be told as the story of how our body matures, selects, releases, and prepares for the arrival of what it hopes is a fertilized egg. When I teach about the menstrual cycle to young girls and their parents, I present a story-based analogy structured around a fictitious "Kingdom." Even though I crafted this story as a way to teach some complicated science to ten-year-old girls, I've had a number of adults tell me that it actually helped them conceptualize the process, too, because they are able to visualize what's happening. So, I want to begin by sharing this story of the Kingdom, because it's a simple foundation for our discussion:

> Imagine a Kingdom that has a very special tradition. Approximately once per month, they invite a Special Guest to come and visit, in the hopes that the Guest will stay. If the Guest arrives and is able to stay with them, the Guest will become the new Prince or Princess of the Kingdom: So you can see that the stakes are fairly high! The people of the Kingdom must work to impress this Guest, so their primary task is to prepare a fabulous guest room fit for royalty.

The uterus is the site of the Kingdom, and the rich endometrium that lines its interior is like the guest room that the other characters work so hard to prepare. The Special Guest is the egg cell, or *ovum,* that is released from the ovary during a menstrual cycle.

As I tell this little story, I teach the girls and their parents

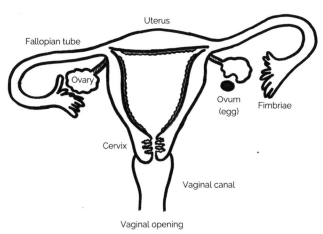

Used with permission from Boston Cross Check, LLC

about the activity of four key hormones throughout various phases of the menstrual cycle: FSH, Estrogen, LH, and Progesterone.

First, FSH (follicle-stimulating hormone) is sent to deliver the invitation to the ovaries that one egg has been selected as this month's Special Guest. This chosen egg should begin to prepare for the great journey toward the Kingdom. The egg develops within a sort of dressing-room called a *follicle* inside the ovary.

Meanwhile, back in the Kingdom (the uterus), Estrogen acts like a Royal Steward and begins carrying out the plans to prepare the Guest Room. Endometrial lining is built up as if Estrogen were furnishing a lavish bed, with luxurious sheets and pillows. At the peak of Estrogen's preparation, FSH goes back to the ovary with its friend, LH (luteinizing hormone), and the two of them signal to the Special Guest that it's time to go! The follicle where the egg had been preparing is now opened — an event called ovulation — and the egg is released from the ovary and begins to travel through the Fallopian tube toward the main part of the uterus.

The follicle now shrivels up and turns into something else within the ovary: It becomes a *corpus luteum*, or a "yellow body," which signals the presence of Progesterone, the Queen hormone.

Under the influence of Progesterone, the Kingdom redoubles its efforts to prepare the Guest Room by making sure the endometrial lining is not only perfectly plush and decadent, but also soft and comforting for the anticipated Guest. But here is where the story gets a little complicated: If, during its journey, the special egg cell has not met up with another special type of cell from a man's body called a *sperm*, then the egg cell will dissolve before it even reaches the Kingdom! So Progesterone and Estrogen and all of the helpers in the Kingdom are not even sure whether the Guest will be arriving or not; and yet they keep working and preparing, just in case.

After enough time has passed and Queen Progesterone is confident there is no Special Guest coming this month, she will instruct the rest of the hormone helpers to clean everything up and get ready to send another invitation. The rich endometrial lining will be shed during an event known as a *period bleed*, and the whole process will start over again.

This story is rather simplified and doesn't provide a perfect analogy, but it helps young girls — and hopefully you, too — begin to think about how events within our bodies are connected. The Kingdom analogy provides the context for understanding all of the important invisible work our bodies do throughout the cycle leading up to a period bleed. While most of us think of the bleed as the key event in our menstrual cycle, because it's the most obvious part, it's actually the release of an egg from its follicle — ovulation — that is the key event.

Our body will continue to go through this cycle from puberty until we reach perimenopause, at which time our hormones start winding down and our body prepares to enter a different sort of fruitfulness after our cycles have stopped. We will reflect more fully on this "reverse puberty" in a later chapter.

For an older audience, we can expand this simplified story to include more background information, because even though we like to speak of the menstrual cycle as a sort of self-contained series of events, that's not quite accurate. Unlike men, whose reproductive cells (sperm) are produced daily throughout the majority of their lives, women's reproductive cells (eggs) are always present in the ovaries in an immature state until "activated" by particular hormones. During each menstrual cycle, many of these follicles actually begin to mature, not just one "Special Guest." But somehow only one is selected to reach full maturity. That selection process is not quite understood yet by science, but even less understood is why our bodies sometimes select two eggs, typically one from each ovary. This is called a double ovulation, and when this happens it means that both ovaries are responding to the same hormonal surges and will release eggs within 24 hours of each other. If both eggs were to be fertilized, this would result in the conception of fraternal twins.

Yet the story is even more complicated because by the time an egg is mature enough to be released at ovulation, it has been developing in its follicle for about ninety to one hundred days. This means that the egg that is released in *this* menstrual cycle actually received its invitation to the Kingdom a few cycles ago.

In other words, our menstrual cycles are not completely self-contained processes. Each cycle is dependent upon the invisible work of previous cycles and will likewise influence the course of the next few cycles as well.

THE UNIQUENESS OF WOMEN'S CYCLES

As someone who spends the majority of her working hours thinking, speaking, and educating on this menstrual cycle, it's odd for me to contemplate how relatively new this knowledge is. We did not even know what mammalian eggs were until 1827, and did not discover the human egg until 1928.[1] This novelty is a concept woven throughout a lot of my thought in these pages, but it's also interesting to note that part of the reason we've been so delayed (relatively speaking) in understanding our menstrual cycles is because we are very different from a lot of other animals, where regular menstruation is fairly uncommon.

The only other known menstruators in the animal kingdom are some apes, a few monkeys, bats, and a couple of other tiny mammals: the elephant shrew and the spiny mouse. The majority of mammals actually undergo a different process called the *estrous cycle*, which is a similar hormonal process but instead of shedding uterine lining, that endometrium is reabsorbed internally. In estrous animals, bleeding signals the period of "heat," when they are ovulating and ready for sexual activity: You may be familiar with this if you have ever owned an unspayed female dog or cat. Because we did not know about this difference, many erroneous theories of fertility persisted for millennia that assumed a woman's most likely chance to conceive was during the time of menstruation. This can be traced back to Aristotle's theories of conception in the fourth century BC, which researchers Bischoff and Pouchet believed they had proved with their discovery of ovulation in the fifteenth century — though they incorrectly assumed that humans were like other animals and ovulated during bleeding days.

When we want to understand anything about our human nature, I think a particular sort of insight can be obtained by asking: "How is this *different* from what we know about the rest of creation? What significance could that have?" We see this same model of inquiry play out in Pope St. John Paul II's *Theology of the Body* through the concept of Original Solitude.

John Paul II asks us to think about the creation of Adam and Eve in the second chapter of Genesis, by pausing to contemplate Adam in the garden *before* Eve is brought forth. Adam, the only human, is tasked by God to seek a suitable companion from the other creatures; so, one by one, Adam calls forth the other animals, comes to know their natures, and gives them names. Throughout this process, one might think that Adam would come to find how similar he is to the other animals and would find a suitable companion from among them, but this is not what happens. Instead, Adam comes to see and understand how different he is from the rest of creation. He realizes that he is a singular sort of creature — an experience John Paul calls *Original Solitude*, which prepares Adam to recognize the great gift of *Original Unity* that he receives in the creation of Eve.

Our menstrual cycles offer women our own experience of Original Solitude, inviting us to see and understand how we are uniquely made, so that we are better prepared to live out the gift of self in motherhood, whether biological or spiritual. It's worth pausing to consider how our menstrual cycles are different from what we find in the rest of the animal kingdom. Is there meaning to be found in our distinction as one of the few menstruator species? Clearly your author thinks the answer is yes, but I'll refrain from commentary at this point and just put forward some of the ways in which we are different:

- Compared with animals that undergo estrus, menstruators experience a relatively hidden ovulation. Our fertility status is not signaled by an attention-grabbing splash of red blood.
- The outermost lining of our endometrium is shed each cycle, rather than being reabsorbed. This means that instead of returning to our body to be used another way, all of the nutrients and energy that were deposited into the building up of the lining are poured forth externally.
- Embryos of menstruators spend the earliest stages of life more physically connected to their mothers than do embryos of non-menstruator mammals. This is because they implant deeper into the uterine lining, into the stroma tissue, instead of into the more superficial top layer of the endometrium.[2]
- Females that undergo estrus are typically only sexually active while in heat, but females with menstrual cycles are known to be sexually active even when they are not ovulating.

You may be thinking: This is interesting, but it's not like humans are totally unique in having menstrual cycles. Other animals do this too, so is it really "unique?" I don't want to insinuate that humans are totally unique in our menstruation, but that this is just one key difference we have from most animals. Original Solitude does not mean coming to understand that every individual aspect about us is completely singular and unique, but rather that we — as a composite and whole creature — are unique. Let's take this observation about the rarity of menstruation and put it into conversation with something I've mentioned before: menopause.

Compared to menstruation in the animal kingdom, menopause is even more rare. Humans, some toothed whales, and chimpanzees are the only species we know of that experience this stage of life. This means that when viewed from the context of our entire reproductive lives, women are very rare in the fact that we both menstruate and go through menopause.

Thus we can see that when we ask the question "What is a menstrual cycle?" our first answer, describing the mere mechanics, is not the whole picture. Once we understand the series of hormonal events that make up a cycle, we are then able to compare this with other animals and see how the menstrual cycle sets us apart within the natural world. And this leads to a fundamental question that seems I've been taking for granted so far, but which bears mentioning and exploration: Are menstrual cycles actually part of God's design for women?

MENSTRUAL CYCLES IN CREATION

The problem we always face when speaking about the body is the nagging question of whether Adam and Eve would have experienced their bodies before the Fall in the same way we experience our bodies here and now.

To sum up a rather complicated teaching: The punishment for Adam and Eve's transgression is a natural consequence of cosmic proportions. As a parent, I know that there are two ways to punish my children when they are misbehaving: I can fabricate some sort of punishment that seems to "fit" the crime (e.g., when I take away the video games because they sat in front of the TV instead of doing their homework), or I can allow them to suffer the natural consequences of their behavior (e.g., I let them fall off the three-foot rock wall I told them for the seventeenth time not to run on). Our collective punishment for going against God falls under the latter category. God basically says, "I'm going to let you experience the effects of what you did. Because you disobeyed me, you are no longer in perfect harmony with your Creator. Because you turned against your own nature, your body and soul are not perfectly in harmony anymore. And because your body and soul are not perfectly in harmony anymore, you are no longer in perfect harmony with the rest of my creation. This means that you will experience death, and you will need to labor in the fields, and you will experience pains in childbirth, and there will be enmity between you and the serpent."[3]

In this book, I'm asking us to reflect on the meaning of our menstrual cycles as they are now, but as Catholics, we also need to think about what these cycles might have looked like in the beginning. In other words, "Did menstrual cycles arise as part of our punishment for sin?"

When we look at the text of Genesis, we learn about the specific implications of original sin for each of the three perpetrators: the serpent, the woman, and the man — in that order. It is worth breaking open the text to focus on this scene, because while the serpent, woman, and man all do have particular consequences associated with their transgressions, there are also deeply relational consequences to their actions. First, God says to the serpent:

> Because you have done this,
>   cursed are you above all cattle,
>   and above all wild animals;
> upon your belly you shall go,
>   and dust you shall eat

> all the days of your life.
> I will put enmity between you and the woman,
>   and between your seed and her seed;
> he shall bruise your head,
>   and you shall bruise his heel. (Genesis 3:14–15)

The first relationship that has been torn asunder is the relationship the serpent has with the other animals. No longer is the serpent one of many — it stands apart as a cursed animal, forced to eat the "dust" upon which all other land animals are privileged to walk. We need not take this literally, but symbolically in the sense that after tricking Adam and Eve, the serpent is now considered a creature set apart from the other creatures through his own guile.

Next, God explains that this creature will now exist in a state of enmity with the woman and her offspring. Note that as of yet, the woman and the man have no offspring. They have been commanded to "Be fruitful and multiply, and fill the earth and subdue it" (Gn 1:28), but that has not yet come to pass. So let us imagine that we are Eve, hearing this speech for the very first time.

Upon hearing the serpent's plight, it is plausible to think that Eve is actually filled with excitement and hope: The promise of offspring has not been denied her! She and Adam will be permitted to carry out their original mission, simply with the addition of a slithery pest nipping at their children. Motherhood is still a promise, even if it will mean a little ingenuity to make sure that her children are safe.

Yet when God turns to the woman, he explains that her motherhood — her relationship with her child — will now be her greatest toil: "I will greatly multiply your pain in childbearing; in pain you shall bring forth children, yet your desire shall be for your husband, and he shall rule over you" (3:16). Yes, motherhood will still be a possibility, but it will not be easy to bring children into this world. And once they are here, they will be threatened at all times by the serpent who seeks to destroy them.

The next relationship to suffer is that of husband and wife, which of course has many implications but would be a topical diversion here. Focusing specifically on the question of menstrual cycles, I believe there are two important things to note in Eve's consequences. The first is that God is very explicit that pains will be associated with childbirth, but the phrase "in pain you shall bring forth children" is open to vast interpretation. Does it specifically mean the pain of labor and birth? Or does it mean that our entire reproductive systems are negatively affected? The wording is not quite clear. Second, even if we take a broad view and assume that the effects of original sin apply to our entire reproductive systems, the only consequence mentioned is pain — God does not explain that he will fabricate an entirely new and torturous way for ovulation to happen. So, I see no necessary reason to assume that the menstrual cycle or even period bleeds would not have been part of God's original design of woman — only that this design would now be susceptible to pain, which was not part of the original plan. We will come back to that point in a moment.

Another question related directly to this conversation: "Did the Blessed Virgin Mary ever have a period?" Through the dogma of the Immaculate Conception, Catholics assert that Mary — like Eve — was born without original sin. In the Church's official proclamation, Pope Pius IX stated, "The Blessed Virgin was, through grace, entirely free from every stain of sin, and from all corruption of body, soul and mind" (*Ineffabilis Deus*). As a result, the harmony she experiences with God is so great that he is able to make himself incarnate in her. Her body and soul are so perfectly united that she did not experience pain in childbirth, and she did not experience death in the same way the rest of us do. Rather than having her body separate from her soul at the end of her earthly life, she was assumed into — taken toward — heaven, both body and soul together. If menstrual cycles were not part of our original design in the Garden, it would seem logical to also conclude that Mary never experienced cycles and period bleeds, either. What are we to make of this?

Since we have no historical record of whether Eve or Mary actually experienced a period bleed, any conclusion we draw on those points must rely on a sort of "fittingness" argument: would it be fitting (or, appropriate and reverent) to say that menstrual cycles were part of our design from the beginning? Let's look at a few facts.

It seems that cycles could be part of our design from the beginning, because God did tell humanity to "be fruitful and multiply" (Gn 1:28), and we need our reproductive systems to do that. The normal, healthy function of the female reproductive system is the menstrual cycle; therefore, it's possible that cycles are part of our original design.

On the other hand, we could speculate that sexual reproduction in the Garden could have happened some other way, without the need for a menstrual cycle. Maybe in the beginning humans were designed to be reflexive ovulators, as we see in many other mammalian species. This would mean that Eve would only ovulate in response to sexual initiation by Adam and — because life was perfect and there was no such thing as miscarriage — she would get pregnant every time and never have a period. That's a possibility, but it requires us to believe in a very big overhaul of an entire body system as a result of original sin. For the sake of consistency, it would also probably force us to say that Adam only ever produced a single, perfect sperm just before sexual intercourse, meaning that his reproductive system would also work very differently from what we know today. St. Edith Stein has summed up the matter most succinctly by stating, "We do not know in what way the blessing of fertility was to be ful-filled in humanity before the Fall."[4]

MAKING SENSE OF CYCLES IN OUR MODERN EXPERIENCE

This is all perhaps interesting to speculate, but for now I consid-er it most prudent to leave the discussion at this: The question of whether Eve experienced a menstrual cycle in the Garden of Eden is an open question in the Church. The faithful are free to explore this question with deference to the Magisterium, and may hold private opinions on the matter without violating any Church teaching.

The fact is that menstrual cycles *as we experience them now* are an intimate aspect of our embodied experience of woman-hood. It is true that for many of us, this experience is riddled with pain and discomfort: It is possible for our menstrual cycles to feel like a sort of disease, or a brokenness that we are expect-ed to live with. But this can be said for any major body system when it is unhealthy. As we will discuss later, these severe sorts of cycle symptoms are not the norm and are actually our body's way of communicating to us that something is very wrong. It can be hard to feel that our cycles are good when they some-times feel so bad, but it's sloppy theology to write off something just because it's not perfect right now. If we did that, we'd have nothing meaningful to say about human nature at all. So, I'd like to take for granted that the onset of our period at menarche, the decades of cycles and bleeds, and the disrupting experience of perimenopause are all the lived theology of our female bodies today. Is it actually constructive and helpful for us to negate or silence that experience only because we're uncomfortable with our understanding of its fittingness?

I believe that an honest exploration into the rich design and meaning of embodied womanhood is going to require us to have positive things to say about our menstrual cycles — regardless of whatever we think our original design may have been. We can take our lead on this going back at least as far as the fourth century, with the compilation document called the *Apostolic Constitutions*. While originally thought to have been a work by Clement of Alexandria, we now suppose an unknown compiler who may have been a bishop. In this document, the compiler gathers together what he believes to be authentic teaching passed on directly from the twelve apostles. In Book VI, there is a specific commentary on sexual prohibitions, which includes this excerpt on menstruation:

> *The fact is that menstrual cycles as we experience them now are an intimate aspect of our embodied experience of womanhood.*

> Therefore neither is the natural purgation abominable before God, who has ordered it to happen to women within the space of thirty days for their advantage and healthful state. ... Nay, moreover, even in the Gospel, when the woman with the perpetual purgation of blood touched the saving border of the Lord's garment in hope of being healed, he was not angry with her, nor did complain of her at all; but, on the contrary, he healed her, saying, "Your faith has saved you."[5]

Very early in our history, we can see that the Church insisted on respect for the healthy, natural function of women's bodies — especially surrounding periods. This should challenge modern women to also consider how our menstrual cycles are part of the way God designed women's health to operate. We are reminded that Jesus does not look down on the woman with a hemorrhage or treat her with disgust: He offers healing for her ailment, just as he welcomed any other sick person who came in search of wholeness. At a minimum, this should show us that devout Catholic women need not consider our cycles and periods to be "curses" in and of themselves.

However, at this point it may seem like we've come to a sort of impasse, where I expect all of my readers to conclude that menstrual cycles were part of God's plan from the beginning. If that were a necessary premise for the rest of this book, anyone who disagrees with that point would find little benefit to this text. So let's consider a sort of "third way," which allows the reader to both remain convinced that cycles and periods were a result of the Fall and still consider cycles and periods to be a good part of our feminine design. To forward that particular view, I'd like to introduce you to a great saint, who is also a Doctor of the Church.

St. Hildegard von Bingen, a twelfth-century abbess, musician, writer, and physician, puts forward the idea that menstrual cycles were not a part of our original design. But instead of being seen as part of Eve's curse, she insinuates that they should still be seen as a blessing. Hildegard lived in a time when blood-letting was seen as a normal part of maintaining health. Her practice of medicine relied heavily on the concept of balancing the "four humors": black bile, yellow bile, phlegm, and blood. It was believed that these four humors were in charge of regulating different aspects of health and personality, and that each person's body must maintain its own unique balance in order to flourish. To ensure that each humor was present in the proper amount, it sometimes was deemed necessary to remove a little bit of blood through small cuts, thereby restoring right proportions and maintaining physical and mental health.

Hildegard posited a very interesting theory in her discussion of periods "Woman has many more noxious humors and much more noxious waste matter in her body than a man…This is evident at the time of menstruation as well. For if she were not purged of noxious humors and waste matter at the time of menstruation, she would swell up completely and become bloated and would not be able to live."[6]

Perhaps you see that word *noxious* and are not quite convinced there is anything positive to be said here, but keep in mind that Hildegard is not making a value judgment. She is articulating the commonly held belief in her time that women did suffer from more imbalance of the humors than men. "Noxious" indicates something harmful or potentially threatening to the health of the person. In Hildegard's understanding, it was precisely the Fall of Adam and Eve in the Garden that first introduced the noxious black bile and thus offset the balance of the humors, bringing sickness into the world.

When viewed in this light, Hildegard's understanding is that even though Eve would not have had a period, our monthly bleeds are not part of the "curse"— they're actually a blessing, which was only given to us as a result of the Fall.

Hildegard does not fully articulate what I am about to explain, but this way of viewing the menstrual cycle actually opens us to an intricate and beautiful understanding of how she thinks God is working in our bodies during a menstrual period. Remember that Hildegard did not understand the process of ovulation and the full menstrual cycle, so she must articulate everything based on how she understands the function of the period bleed itself. What she believes is that periods are the natural way a woman's body rids itself of these "noxious imbalances." In other words, they are the way God has designed our bodies for the process of natural bloodletting. Left on its own after the Fall, Hildegard says that the female body would be so filled with bile that it would basically poison itself in fairly short order. God — perhaps Hildegard could say "The Divine Bloodletter" — did not want woman to suffer the natural consequence of the transgression in the Garden with all of those noxious humors as a result. So, God blessed women with a monthly bloodletting to maintain her physical and mental health.

When viewed in this light, Hildegard's understanding is that even though Eve would not have had a period, our monthly bleeds are not part of the "curse"— they're actually a *blessing,* which was only given to us as a result of the Fall.

Lest that you think your author has gotten a little too fanciful, such a conclusion is not particularly far-fetched. We do have Biblical support that God has done this sort of thing before. After Cain's heinous fratricide, God condemns him to the life of wandering the earth:

> Cain said to the Lord, "My punishment is greater than I can bear. Behold, you have driven me this day away from the ground; and from your face I shall be hidden; and I shall be a fugitive and a wanderer on the earth, and whoever finds me will slay me." Then the Lord said to him, "Not so! If any one slays Cain, vengeance shall be taken on him sevenfold." And the Lord put a mark on Cain, lest any who came upon him should kill him. (Genesis 4:13–15)

The mark given to Cain was actually a sign of God's blessing: Even though God still made Cain experience the consequences of his sin, he did not allow Cain to suffer them to the full extent. St. Ambrose of Milan suggests that through this mark, God offered Cain a twofold mercy: First, that Cain would not be killed by another person, and second, that Cain would have time on earth for repentance: "As regards the token God placed on Cain with the purpose of protecting him from death at the hands of another, this may be said. He wanted the wanderer to have time for reflection and by such kindness inspire him to change his ways."[7]

In other words, the mark of Cain is an active intervention from God that preserves Cain from suffering the full extent of his crime (death), and even creates a new opportunity for Cain to be reconciled with God. For Hildegard, therefore, it seems that periods are a parallel to the mark of Cain: God actively gives us menstrual bleeds to preserve women from suffering the full extent of the natural consequences of Eve's crime, which would have been death. By Hildegard's account, we can imagine that both Adam and Eve would have felt and understood the introduction of this new, noxious black bile into their biology. Yet Eve's response would have been more dire than Adam's, because she knew of her own weakness. Like Cain, Eve would cry out to God: "My punishment is greater than I can bear! Behold, I shall surely die before I am able to bring forth my offspring!" Thus the Lord created the natural purgation of blood, lest the swelling and bloating of bile should kill her. Hildegard, therefore, seems to believe that periods were not something women would have experienced if we had remained in Eden, yet God has provided them to be healthful and good in our current state.

The fact that Hildegard was working with very limited biology should not deter us from this conclusion that periods are healthy and good for women. This is precisely the starting point that I would like all modern women and girls to be able to embrace. Even if periods are difficult, and even if we are convinced that this was *not* how things were supposed to be in the beginning, we are still invited to consider what it might mean for our cycles to be a form of blessing. We are invited to ponder why our God gave us this unique process. We'll continue exploring this question together throughout this book.

CHAPTER 2

Why Should the Church Care about Cycles?

Before we reflect more deeply on the meaning of women's cycles, it is worth asking whether the Church should actually care about the topic in the first place. After all, I've never seen a book about the theological significance of auditory processing. I'm not sure that anyone ever read Jesus' words "He who has ears to hear, let him hear" (Mt 11:15) and thought to themselves, "I wonder what the structure of the inner ear and its connection to the auditory cortex can tell us about Jesus' exhortations to hear." Maybe someone should write that book ... this is, after all, what the theological concept of mystery is all about — we can never exhaust the meaningful ways to explore who God is, and who we are in relation to him as creatures. But there is something special about menstrual cycles compared with other body systems, and that something special merits exploration in the Church.

To be clear: By "the Church" I do not mean the bishops and priests and moral theologians. Or rather, I do not *exclusively* mean the bishops and priests and moral theologians. Saint Paul reminds us that all the baptized are members of the Body of Christ, which is the Church (see Rom 12; 1 Cor 12), meaning that when we speak of the need for "the Church" to do something, we include every single member who has been given the gifts to assist with that particular need. Yes, we desperately need the leadership of our clergy to teach and encourage couples to live out the Church's theology of marriage and sex — but even more than that, we desperately need the expertise and the willingness of lay people to walk with one another. We need women to step up in holy boldness and ask tough questions about this often-maligned part of our female bodies.

BECAUSE CYCLES ARE PART OF WOMAN'S BIOLOGY

In the first place, women, as members of the Body of Christ, deserve to have our bodies respected in their entirety, in *all* of their functions. As a Church, we have beautiful meditations on how some functions of the female body echo the presence and working of God. Our tradition passes on a rich set of theology and imagery surrounding pregnancy, childbirth, and child-rearing. The Akathist Hymn, a sixth-century prayer in honor of the Virgin Mary, shows how a woman's womb is like a tabernacle: "By singing praise to your maternity, we all exalt you as a spiritual temple, Mother of God! For the One Who Dwelt Within Your Womb, the Lord Who Holds All Things in His Hands, sanctified you, glorified you, and taught all men to sing to you: Hail, O Tabernacle of God the Word!" This applies to Mary in a particular way as the biological Mother of God, but by extension we can meditate on how every woman's womb, when it carries a child, is like a tabernacle in which the *image* of the Divine quietly dwells.

We can also reflect on the nourishment women's bodies can give to our children in the various ways God speaks to Israel like a tender mother. In Genesis 17, God even calls himself *El Shaddai*, which can literally be translated as "mighty teat," or perhaps more poetic to our modern Western sensibilities, "the Almighty One who nourishes us."

These are merely a glimpse into the rich theology of the Church around women's bodies; yet while we focus so much on what the female body can do for others, we seldom talk about what the female body symbolizes in and of itself. It is true that the menstrual cycle is associated with these other functions of pregnancy, birth, and nourishment because cycles are ordered toward procreation, as we saw in the previous chapter. But why are they not mentioned? Everything the menstrual cycle does is at the service of creating an environ-

> *Women, as members of the Body of Christ, deserve to have our bodies respected in their entirety, in all of their functions.*

ment where pregnancy is possible, so it does seem an odd omission that our theology has not expressed the same reverence for cycles as it does for pregnancy. Perhaps that omission is simply due to a historical lack of information, in which case now seems an appropriate time to explore this topic in earnest!

Yet, a woman's purpose on this earth is not simply procreation. Like men, we are created to become saints. We are made to be holy, whether or not we ever have biological children. Thus, when we reflect on the teachings of the Church regarding motherhood, women may sometimes end up feeling a bit adrift. If we only are given the tools and the imagery to meditate about our bodies in their biological function *for the other,* we can end up grasping for meaning when we aren't performing that specific function. And as much as we can and should talk about the rich meaning of spiritual motherhood, that doesn't erase the fact that spiritual mothers bleed from their physical bodies.

In the next chapter, we will look deeper at the importance of human bodies as part of the way men and women image God; but here it makes sense to mention that our Church is able to have a rich theology about certain bodily functions precisely because humans are body-soul creatures. The *Catechism of the Catholic Church* states, "The human person, created in the image of God, is a being at once corporeal and spiritual" (362), and "the unity of soul and body is so profound that one has to consider the soul to be the 'form' of the body" (365). Therefore, there should be a relationship between respecting the biology of a person's body and reverencing the person as a whole. The Church thus has an invitation to deepen our theology of "woman" by looking at the biology of menstrual cycles and period bleeds, beginning with the concept that cycles are integral to women's health.

When we go to the doctor's office, most of us are familiar with the concept of "vital signs": the four key indicators of overall health that are usually measured even before the doctor will come to see you. These indicators are temperature, blood pressure, heart rate, and breathing rate. A fifth sign of "pain level" is often also included as a vital piece of information. Yet the American College of Obstetricians and Gynecologists has added an additional vital sign for girls: the menstrual cycle.[1] Their majority committee opinion, written in 2015 and reaffirmed in 2020, clearly states: "It is important for clinicians to have an understanding of the menstrual patterns of adolescent girls, the ability to differentiate between normal and abnormal menstruation, and the skill to know how to evaluate the adolescent girl patient. By including an evaluation of the menstrual cycle as an additional vital sign, clinicians reinforce its importance in assessing overall health status for patients and caretakers."

This medical opinion has nothing to do with cycles as a vital sign relating to fertility. It has nothing to do with reproductive function. It is a statement, endorsed by the American Academy of Pediatrics, that insists that menstrual cycles themselves are crucial to understanding and addressing the health of female patients. In other words, clinicians are seeing that cycles are not just important for understanding a woman's fertility. Cycles are important for understanding a woman.

In *Mulieris Dignitatem*, John Paul II writes about the need for us to seriously consider what we know in this day and age about the bio-physiological and psychological processes of conception, pregnancy, and birth. But he clarifies:

> What the different branches of science have to say on this subject is important and useful, provided that it is not limited to an exclusively bio-physiological interpretation of women and of motherhood. Such a "restricted" picture would go hand in hand with a materialistic concept of the human being and of the world. In such a case, what is truly essential would unfortunately be lost. (18)

Christians must always respect and consider the truths of science. Truth, no matter where it is found, has its origin in God himself. Science is a mode of natural revelation. But we must always guard against the temptation to solely focus on the materialistic truth about the human body; instead we must focus on the whole truth of the human person. The Church in this day and age needs to think about the growing body of knowledge surrounding menstrual cycle science and consider how it might impact both our theology of "woman" in a broad sense, and our pastoral care of women who deeply yearn for better ways to understand the dignity of their female bodies.

BECAUSE CYCLES ARE OFTEN
PLACES OF SUFFERING

The Church must also contend seriously with the fact that sometimes women's cycles and periods are painful. Sometimes they are a source of real trauma in our bodies; and if we take seriously what the Church teaches about the unity of soul and body, we must consider that physical pain is often also a deeply spiritual pain. Too often I have noticed a tendency to dismiss period pain because it is just assumed as a "normal" part of woman's existence; but this is not reflective of our Church's stance on suffering in general. And, if hard-pressed, I do not think any serious theologian would insist that pain in our uterus should be treated any less seriously than pain anywhere else. So why does our Church not speak of these issues in the same way we speak of other pain and suffering?

A full survey of the Church's teaching on suffering, pain, and the existence of evil would be impossible in this text. Yet, there are a few core things we should keep in mind as we consider menstrual cycles and their relationship to suffering and pain. First, we know that suffering and death entered this world as a result of humanity's transgression in the Garden of Eden. God did not intend for us to suffer the effects of evil in our bodies, but humanity rejected God's will in favor of our own. Next, in order to free us from death, sin, and suffering, the Eternal Son of God became incarnate in the person of Jesus of Nazareth. John Paul II explains, "even though the victory over sin and death achieved by Christ in his Cross and Resurrection does not abolish temporal suffering from human life, nor free from suffering the whole historical dimension of human existence, it nevertheless throws a new light upon this dimension and upon every suffering: the light of salvation," (*Salvifici Doloris*, 15). In other words, Christ makes it possible for our own sufferings to be united with his in the work of salvation and, through this union, to actually be drawn closer and more intimately to God. This is the key to embracing suffering as redemptive, and offering up our sufferings willingly to Christ.

Yet, our moments of suffering are also an invitation for others to become the loving, healing hands of Christ in our lives. John Paul II goes on to say that "suffering, which is present under so many different forms in our human world, is also present in order to unleash love in the human person" (29). So we are not meant to suffer alone, in silence; our personal sufferings are meant to be communicated to and received by others so that others may become more like Christ in his merciful love and compassion. This is a delicate balance to preserve, but we see it play out both in the parable of the Good Samaritan and directly in Jesus' own healing ministry.

In Luke's Gospel, we read about a particular healing account that will come up multiple times in our discussions on cycles: the healing of the woman with a hemorrhage: "And a woman who had had a flow of blood for twelve years and had spent all her living upon physicians and could not be healed by any one, came up behind him, and touched the fringe of his garment; and immediately her flow of blood ceased" (Lk 8:43–44).

According to Mosaic law, this woman was unclean and therefore unfit to have contact with another human being for *twelve years.* Jesus attributes her healing to the power of her faith, but we can also sense the desperation in this healing. She has spent all of her money. She has had no relief. She is anemic, in pain, and oh so tired. This woman senses that when Jesus walks by, there is healing to be found; her faith manifests as realized hope that this, at last, is the Divine Physician she has longed for all these years. She boldly reaches out to seek healing and receives it.

When we read this account, the woman's plight almost tempts us to incredulity: *Twelve years??? That's absurd!* But the average time in the United States today for a woman to receive a diagnosis of endometriosis is currently about seven to eight years. I worry that this delay is not just due to ignorance of symptoms or inherent issues with the medical system, but also because women have internalized this idea that our cycles are not worthy of healing. I have had conversations with other women about my work, and in more than a handful of cases I have been told that "We shouldn't lie to girls about their periods being good. Periods are just painful and a part of life they can't control. We need to teach them how to suck it up and deal."

If Catholic women don't have any meaningful way to claim their cycles and periods as good, then we have cornered ourselves into silence. When we see cycles and periods as an inconvenient "add on" to an embodied female living in this world, if we have nothing positive to say about this crucial aspect of our bodies, the natural consequence is that women will not seek healing. And while we can certainly grow in virtue and encounter Christ in suffering, we must remember that the goal in life is not to suffer as much as we possibly can — otherwise Christ would not call us to help alleviate the suffering of others, nor would he have worked any healing miracles by his own hands or allow his saints to do the same. We deserve to have that same faith and confidence in our Divine Physician as the woman in Luke's Gospel. We deserve to feel that God wills our healing. We deserve to know that our body, in all of its functions, is loved and cared for by Christ.

All this is to say, there are deep theological reasons why a woman, as a member of the Body of Christ, would want to include her menstrual cycles in her understanding of the goodness of her body. Where else can she find this but in her Catholic faith, which alone holds this tension between claiming the body as part of the goodness of creation, without downplaying the real suffering that is associated with embodied life?

BECAUSE CYCLES ARE PART
OF FAMILY PLANNING

When people typically think about reasons the Church should care about menstrual cycles, Natural Family Planning is probably the first — and sometimes the only — reason that comes to mind. It's true: The Church needs to talk about menstrual cycles because this is the practical information couples need in order to practice Natural Family Planning. Apart from total abstinence, NFP is the only method of regulating births that the Church supports. So, the Catholic Church quite literally requires couples to learn about and consider menstrual cycles in a way and to a degree that she does not require for other body systems. In fact, Poper Paul VI states that this knowledge is a requirement for responsible parenthood, regardless of whether or not the couple will discern the need to postpone or space pregnancies:

> Married love, therefore, requires of husband and wife the full awareness of their obligations in the matter of responsible parenthood, which today, rightly enough, is much insisted upon, but which at the same time should be rightly understood. Thus, we do well to consider responsible parenthood in the light of its varied legitimate and interrelated aspects.
>
> With regard to the biological processes, responsible parenthood means an awareness of, and respect for, their proper functions. In the procreative faculty the human mind discerns biological laws that apply to the human person. (*Humanae Vitae*, 10)

Perhaps, by way of experiment, we can imagine a world in which the Church does not need to provide any of the practical knowledge to women or couples about cycles. Maybe in this counterfactual world, we would have a society that freely shares this valuable information with girls as soon as they begin menstruating, by teaching them how to observe and chart their cycles with an eye toward understanding and respecting their natural bodily functions as they grow. We can imagine in this world that artificial hormones, which override natural cycles and create artificial period bleeds, would not be a standard cure-all treatment for teen cycle issues. Girls would instead understand what normal and atypical variations are in their cycles, and would be able to ask for help from trusted adults when they notice patterns of concern.

This wonderful world would require that all healthcare professionals have at least a basic understanding of the changing phases and particular biomarkers of hormonal activity in the woman's menstrual cycle. Doctors would have accurate representation of efficacy rates for NFP on their family planning options poster, and be willing to recommend it — or at least support a patient's choice to use it — at any point during a woman's reproductive life. Teens would share charting knowledge with their peers. Adult friends would speak casually and comfortably about their preferred NFP method, recommending favorite instructors or reading materials as enthusiastically as they might recommend their favorite mechanic or hair stylist. In this imaginary world, a Catholic couple would have all of the social, educational, and medical support they needed in order to consider these biological processes of responsible parenthood, requiring only minimal pastoral support from their parish.

But notice that even in this imaginary world, where the parish is only called upon to form and support the couple according to the virtuous exercise of responsible parenthood, the Church still needs to understand the particulars of what NFP entails! A priest who thinks that couples only need to abstain for six days each cycle will not understand or be able to offer practical help to the woman who confesses again and again that she struggles with abstinence. A men's group full of guys who don't understand the complexity of fertility biomarkers and differences among NFP methods will not be prepared to comfort a new dad who is anxious about another unexpected pregnancy.

Sex and parenthood are part of the core mystery of how marriage itself images God, because these physical realities point to the truth that God's mysterious Triune communion of persons bears fruit within itself. The image of father, mother, and child — the earthly trinity — comes about through sex and parenthood. Much theological reflection in the Church invites us to dive into this great mystery and to see the Sacrament of Matrimony itself as another layer of God's mysterious life: his union with his own creatures through the marriage of Christ and the Church.

All of this is beautiful and inspiring to those whose hearts are inclined to hear the Good News of sex and marriage. But we live in a society that treats sex as little more than entertainment, and children as an opt-in facet of one's adult lifestyle. It's time for the Church — for all of us — to step in and step up to correct these misunderstandings. It's also incumbent upon the Church to provide sound pastoral support for couples who sincerely desire children but experience infertility and have a difficult time seeing how their family of two has a place in the Body of Christ.

For these and many more pastoral reasons, the Church needs to be serious about helping couples understand the biological dimension of responsible parenthood. We need to be a community where couples can reliably find, and expect that their fellow parishioners understand, basic information about how this particular aspect of our bodies works. This kind of community allows us to be concrete about ways that husbands and wives can grow in the graces, virtues, and duties presented to them in the Sacrament of Matrimony.

BECAUSE THE WORLD IS CONFUSED ABOUT BODIES

But the reality is that my wonderful, counterfactual world does not exist. Many women and men do not have easy access to information about cycles and family planning outside of what they find in the Church. It is not yet standard practice for doctors to include menstrual cycle charting as part of their diagnosis and treatment plans for women. Despite growing interest, NFP still remains such a relatively uncommon practice that women and men do not often find support from friends or family. I try to be generous in my assumptions and think that most doctors or educators are either simply unaware of the importance of menstrual cycles to women's health or are too busy to learn about it. But a closer look at our current culture seems to indicate that the world is not merely ignorant of but often downright hostile to this aspect of women's biology.

> *Our modern dualist heresy attacks not just the body, but the meaningful difference between female and male bodies.*

The entire birth control industry is built around the lie that fertility is a burden, rather than a blessing. We are told that sex should be for pleasure and entertainment, so what we do with our bodies doesn't matter as long as it makes us happy. This is not the Catholic understanding of fertility, sex, marriage, and family. This is not how Catholics understand the inherent dignity of the body and the fact that the things we do with our bodies affect our souls. In short, this is our job as a Church, because we are the only ones right now who are equipped to do it.

Yet you might wonder how I can propose that the Church *needs* to provide education and support on this topic, since it's a relatively new area of science. After all, for the vast majority of human history and Church history, we have not been able to explore family planning and responsible parenthood sufficiently in the biological dimension. Cycles themselves have not been understood until relatively recently in modern medicine, and we are still discovering many things about them. How can something that seems to be novel in the modern era be required of the Church?

I'd like to posit that it is precisely the uniqueness of our current time that now places this responsibility on the Church. While there are no new heresies under the sun, the lies of the evil one do present themselves in novel ways, and one very ancient heresy called *dualism* is rearing its ugly head today in a unique way. The core belief of dualism is that the whole material world is somehow evil, and that matter itself is therefore an obstacle to the pure, spiritual life that God designed for us.

This heresy was seen clearly in the very early Church with Marcion, who put together his own canon of Scripture that included only a modified set of the Pauline Epistles and an abbreviated version of the Gospel of Luke. Marcion taught that the "God" of the Old Testament was actually a Demiurge, a tribal deity of the Jewish people who was responsible for creating the material world. He contrasted this Demiurge with the Father of Jesus Christ, whom Marcion claimed to be the true God. This God did not actually become incarnate in the material world — no, that would be an obscenity. Instead, Marcion explained that Jesus put on the *appearance* of matter in order to preach the existence of the One True God.

A similar belief was put forward by Mani in the third century, who saw himself as the final prophet of the truth, preaching the fullness of what Jesus began to teach. The core tenant of this dualism is the fight between the World of Darkness and the World of Light, played out between matter (which, according to Mani, is evil) and the pure goodness of spirit. This was the sect to which Saint Augustine belonged as a young man, and was the same heresy that returned in twelfth-century France through the Albigenses. As a Lay Dominican, I owe much of my spiritual heritage to the Church's response to this particular group, because it was precisely to combat the Albigenses that Saint Dominic took up his preaching ministry.

Modern-day Christianity even has residual hints of dualism sprinkled throughout: One of my biggest annoyances about popular theology in America today is the mistaken belief that when a person dies and goes to heaven, they get their angel wings. "Heaven gained another angel today" is a common sentiment offered to a friend suffering the loss of a loved one. The underlying message is intended to comfort those left behind, but the legacy of this strange idea is almost total cultural amnesia about the universal resurrection. Heaven is not a place where happy spirits of dead people fly around with wings and harps — it is the place where the souls of the just experience the beatific vision and await the final consummation of God's promise for a New Jerusalem. This popular image of people-turned-angels not only insults the nature and purpose of angels as God's cosmic agents, but it reeks of confusion about what it means to actually be a *human,* to be a body-soul creature made in the image and likeness of God.

It should come as no surprise that dualism, this outright attack on the material existence of humankind, is a favorite repeat tactic of the devil. The devil hates the material of the world, and in a particular way the devil hates the material of our bodies, because he abhors the fact that God chose to become incarnate and dwell with us as a human. He hates that there is a human Queen of heaven and is jealous of the love God has for us, particularly, as creatures. This is not new, and until the New Jerusalem is fully realized, it will be a constant battle that the Church is called to fight.

But here, I believe, is precisely where the Church needs to take up the unique "weapon" of menstrual cycle science and fertility awareness, because our modern dualist heresy attacks not just the body, but the meaningful difference between female and male bodies. Our society now generally holds the notion that our bodies are so completely inconsequential to our identities that a person could *be* something other than what they physically are — that a person could be a "man trapped in a woman's body" or vice versa, without anything meaningful to say about what it means to be a "woman" if you don't have a biologically female body.

On one level, we can see how thoughtful Catholics might actually resonate with this idea, because we have what appears to be an example of this phenomenon in the Eucharist. In the Blessed Sacrament, the appearance is that of bread and wine, but the substance is actually the body and blood, soul and divinity of Jesus Christ. Could it not be the case that a similar reality may be at play within the person who experiences gender dysphoria? Setting aside the necessary social and cultural analysis of the current transgender movement, we can admit that persistent gender dysphoria is a real issue that a very small number of people do experience. I have a deep sympathy for those who suffer greatly through feeling that their body and their soul are somehow not quite "together." This is a profoundly and uniquely human way to suffer, because there is no other creature that is even capable of suffering in this particular way. Angels do not have bodies and animals do not possess rational souls; we humans are the only sort of creature who could possibly feel a tension between our body (exterior) and our soul (interior).

But here is where any attempted parallel with the Eucharist breaks down, because God is a completely different species from both bread and wine. When God enters into the Eucharist, the substance of bread and wine no longer exist. The Eucharist is something completely new: the substance of Christ's body, blood, soul, and divinity … just with the appearance, or *accidents*, of bread and wine. When we understand, as the Church teaches, that to be human is to be both body and soul together, we see that neither the body nor the soul can be considered a "species" of its own. They cannot be separated in this way, and so there is no meaningful way to say that I *am* something other than what my body-soul composite is.

This is precisely why I like to focus on menstrual cycles and why I believe they are so crucial for the Church to explore in this moment: They are a physical manifestation of the strange mystery of "womanhood." Philosophical and even theological discussions about the abstract meaning of *woman* are certainly interesting, but I often feel uncomfortable with them. If womanhood could be summed up in a few particular virtues or inclinations of the soul, then any person who exhibited those virtues or inclinations would be a woman. In that case, it seems that we could talk meaningfully about a "woman trapped in a man's body" and vice versa. But to the Christian, this does not make sense.

I remember speaking with a friend many years ago, who was truly struggling with the Church's teaching that only men can be priests. I explained that one reason, perhaps the biggest reason, is that Christ himself was a man. When he sat with his friends at the Last Supper, he did so in a male body. And so during the Mass, when the priest acts *in persona Christi,* it must be a man. In the same way we need the proper matter of wine and bread to confect the Eucharist, we need a man to stand in the place of Christ because that is the proper matter for the sacrament.

She looked at me and winced a little. "But …" she chose her words very carefully, "it's just so … *physical.*"

And that, right there, is what we must contend with as Catholic Christians. We must face the fact that our religion does not allow us *not* to be physical. But we must also face the fact that our religion does not allow us to be *merely* physical.

With so much confusion, discomfort, and outright rejection

of the nature of the human person in our world today, it falls to the Church to reawaken humanity to the reality of our creaturehood. In the pages that follow, we will first embark upon an exploration of how menstrual cycles, as part of woman's embodied existence, deepen our understanding of the way women uniquely image God. We will then propose a few concrete ways that growing in knowledge and appreciation for this aspect of woman's biology can deepen our relationship with God, with others, and with ourselves as beloved daughters of God. By laying this groundwork, we will be able to counter the lies and errors of modern dualism and — as a Church — better serve women and couples in these important areas of wholeness, healing, family planning, and holiness.

CHAPTER 3

Menstrual Cycles in the Female *Imago Dei*

In the second half of this book, we will take what we know about the biology of menstrual cycles and ask questions such as: How can knowing this about my body help me become more *myself?* How could knowing this about myself help me understand God better? How could this knowledge serve me in my pursuit of holiness? But before we enter that discussion, I'd like to lay some theological groundwork, because most of us have never been invited to see our menstrual cycles as something that can give us positive knowledge about ourselves or about God.

So, over the next few chapters, we are going to explore various ways in which our menstrual cycles contribute to our understanding of how women uniquely image God.

WHAT DOES IT MEAN TO BE MADE IN GOD'S IMAGE?

Scripture tells us that in the beginning, God created both man and woman together, both equally sharing in his image and likeness. "So God created man in his own image, in the image of God he created him; male and female he created them" (Gn 1:27). The shorthand Latin we use for this is *imago Dei*, which means simply "the image of God." No other creature, not even the angels, was given this same dignity. Nor was any other creature given the dual existence that humanity experiences: to be an embodied rational soul is, as far as we know, completely unique in all the rest of creation. So, what does this unique status of *imago Dei* mean for us?

In part, the *imago Dei* is about how our soul reflects certain aspects of God. Lesson 5 from the *Baltimore Catechism*[1] explains:

> **48. What is man?**
> Man is a creature composed of body and soul, and made to the image and likeness of God.
> *And God created man to his own image. (Genesis 2:7)*

> **49. Is this likeness to God in the body or in the soul?**
> This likeness to God is chiefly in the soul.

> **50. How is the soul like God?**
> The soul is like God because it is a spirit having understanding and free will, and is destined to live forever.
> *And the dust return into its earth, from whence it was, and the spirit return to God, who gave it. (Ecclesiastes 12:7)*

Taking "man" to collectively mean both male and female, we can see how the human person in both sexes equally images God through these aspects of understanding, free will, and the capacity for eternal life with God.

Yet notice that the catechism says "chiefly" in the soul — not exclusively. The angels also have understanding, free will, and the chance to spend eternal life with God, and yet they are not made in his image. We cannot neglect the other aspect of our human nature, the body, which must somehow be a part of the way we image God.

One way our bodies participate in the *imago Dei* is the fact that male and female bodies are capable of coming together as a communion of persons. As Christians, we understand that God is a triune entity — three persons, in perfect union with one another as one God. Pope St. John Paul II explains:

> Man becomes an image of God not so much in the moment of solitude as in the moment of communion. He is, in fact, "from the beginning" not only an image in which the solitude of one Person … but also and essentially the image of an inscrutable divine communion of Persons. (*Thelogy of the Body* 9:3)

The most obvious way physical communion is achieved is through the act of sexual intercourse, the moment when the sexual differences of our bodies make the most sense. In some cases, this sexual union will result in the creation of new human life, meaning that this particular union of man and woman is also capable of imaging God through biological fruitfulness. In Genesis 1:28, God's first command to the man and woman is: "'Be fruitful and multiply.'" From the beginning, our complementarity was placed at the service of life, and in this way, male and female bodies image the creative relationships between the persons of the Trinity: the Spirit proceeds from the relationship between the Father and the Son. Of course, sexual complementarity and biological fruitfulness are not the only way humanity images God; but they are perhaps the most immediate and intelligible illustration of this capacity for communion through which *imago Dei* is expressed.

We've established how our souls image God, and how the unity of man and woman images God. Can we also say that individual bodies image God? The answer here must be unequivocally yes! The Church explains that one way this is accomplished is through the dimension of "sign" or "sacramentality" that God has chosen for this world. Invisible spiritual realities do not remain hidden in the visible world, but are actually represented or made manifest through physical matter. In other words, our physical bodies function as a visible *sign* of the invisible God, in whose image we are made. This means that through the matter of a man's body and the matter of a woman's body, God allows us to better understand him by way of analogy — applying some aspect of our physical bodies to the spiritual nature of God.

> *In other words, our physical bodies function as a visible sign of the invisible God, in whose image we are made.*

Scripture is rich with this sort of imagery: When Mary proclaims "He has shown strength with his arm" (Lk 1:51), she is, of course, not speaking of God's literal arm. She means that God's power is like an arm, which deals mighty blows. When the Psalmist sings, "Your right hand supported me" (Ps 18:36), he does not speak of God's literal right hand, but of God's favor for his chosen people.

The saints also engage in this style of theology. In her *Book of Divine Works,* St. Hildegard von Bingen explains how we can proceed by analogy from the unique structure of the human body to understand certain characteristics of God:

> In the nostrils, God signifies wisdom, which is the fra-

grant observance of order in all skills, so that, by its fragrance, a person may recognize what wisdom ordains. For the sense of smell is diffused widely among all creatures, drawing in their scents so that a person may know what they are like. By the mouth, God designates his Word through which he created all things, just as everything is spoken by the mouth with the sound of rationality. For a person utters many things by speaking, just as the Word of God, creating in the embrace of love, arranged that nothing necessary should be lacking to his work. And just as the cheeks and chin surround the mouth, so the beginning of all creation was present to the Word when it sounded, when all things were created; and thus in the beginning was the Word.[2]

Saint Basil takes up a similar project in his discourses on the Divine Image, saying:

Effort has been spent in much diligent study of the human body that belongs to all of us. If you study medicine, you will find how many things it describes to us, how many hidden vessels it has discovered in our internal structure through anatomical dissection, tunnels in the invisible, a single confluence of the body, the channels of breath, the pipelines of blood, the drawing of breath, the dwelling of a hearth of heat by the heart, the continuous movement of breath around the heart. There are thousands of observations concerning these things with which no one of us is acquainted, for nobody has the leisure to take on this field of research, neither does each know himself as he is … "Wonderful is your knowledge from me," and the craftsmanship that is in me, understanding by what wisdom my body is structured. From this small work of construction, I understand the great Fashioner.[3]

Of course, coming to know God through analogy is an imperfect method. Whenever we want to say that one particular quality or another is *like* an aspect of God, we have to remember that it is even more *unlike* God — simply because God is a mystery far beyond our understanding. So if we say God is *like* a human mother, we also have to know that God is very much *unlike* a human mother because a human mother is inherently finite and limited. This should not stop us, however, from using the language of sign to delve into reflection on particular aspects of God through his image, written into our bodies.

MEDITATION ON THE BODY AS A PATH TO KNOWLEDGE

When we understand that our bodies are meant to signify something about God, then the task is left for us to ask: What do they signify? What can I learn about myself and about God by better understanding my physical body as part of God's image?

It may seem odd at first to consider how our menstrual cycles image God because the fact is that many women do suffer through very difficult experiences with cycles and periods. Pain, shame, embarrassment, illness, or the cross of infertility may all lead us to think that our cycles and periods are things of the devil, rather than our good, loving Father. Yet those experiences of physical and psychological evil through our cycles are not constitutive of our cycles themselves; they are a result of our bodies living in this fallen world. Therefore, the more we can do to dive deeper into understanding our design and biology as women, the more clearly we will be able to discern the beauty and goodness of God's design amidst the messiness of everything else.

This idea that the science of biology can help us better understand God is not limited to our cycles, of course, because female biology cannot be limited to a single function. But neither should cycles be excluded from our meditation on woman, because they are so fundamental to our biology.

Bl. Nicholas Steno, a seventeenth-century Danish scientist and bishop, believed that all study of science was a valid launching point for meditation on God, but especially biology, because "This is the true purpose of anatomy: to lead the audience by the wonderful artwork of the human body to the dignity of the soul and by the admirable structure of both to the knowledge and love of God."[4] This sort of understanding of the relationship between the natural world, humans, and God is what is commonly referred to as the "pedagogy of creation," the process by which observing the works of God can lead us to deeper understanding of ourselves as creatures, and ultimately of God himself.

We can imagine an analogy in which creation is like a great painting. Even within the same style and period, individual artists have recognizable differences. They can have unique ways of playing with shapes and light, or easily recognizable brushstroke patterns. Learning about and paying attention to these sorts of details not only help us to identify who the artist is when the authenticity of a piece of artwork may be in question, but they can even be an interesting window into the artist herself. In a similar fashion, we can look at creation and ask ourselves, "What does this fabulous work tell me about God?"

This process through which we learn about the Creator by observing the creature is supremely heightened when it comes to people, because we were made differently from everything else.

I like to think of all of the rest of creation as a beautiful landscape — but the creation of the human person is like God's self-portrait. It's how God would depict himself using the media of "body" and "soul." So when we look at the form of the human person — even down to the level of body systems and cellular structure — we can see that as an invitation from God to use that as a point of reflection and meditation on himself.

EMBRACING GOD'S IMAGE IN THE FEMALE BODY

We have already touched on the fact that women's bodies image God through their relationship to men's bodies and the procreative potential that coupling holds. This is what John Paul II often refers to in his *Theology of the Body* as "Original Unity." But our task for the rest of this book will be to contemplate the uniqueness of a woman's body in itself, rather than exclusively focusing on woman's relationship to man.

There is a wisdom to this, as St. Teresa Benedicta of the Cross (Edith Stein) explains: "The meaning of the specifically feminine being is not to be understood only in relation to man … Moreover, it has already been emphasized that all creatures related to God in their divine likeness; thus it is befitting the feminine nature that her characteristic function is to reflect the divine."[5]

Woman's identity as *imago Dei* is a higher and more fundamental identity than any other part of ourselves. If we fail to recognize God's image living in our very bodies, then we will be hard-pressed to understand or appreciate any of the other roles we play in life, even those beautiful vocational roles of wife, religious sister, or consecrated virgin.

I am keenly aware, however, that it can be difficult for women to really sit and think about how our bodies are *like* God. God doesn't have personal, firsthand experience of living as a woman in the same way he experienced life as a man. Jesus was — and remains — a male human, and this is re-presented to us each time we see a male priest. At times, this has made me feel as if my own type of body was somehow undesirable for God to inhabit, or that God does not want to be *with me* in my womanhood in the same way he is *with* men.

If that is where you find yourself, then let me affirm you in that tension. It's okay to have questions and to explore them with God, as long as this is done in a spirit of humility, and we are truly seeking understanding. In many ways, that's precisely what the rest of this text is meant to do: to give women the space to open up very raw and honest conversations with ourselves and with God about this aspect of our biology that is so often maligned in our culture. To me, it feels very primal, earthy, and tangible to ask God directly: In what way does my menstrual cycle *image* You?

To dive into that question, we will first look at some qualities of God that are already expressed symbolically through circles and cycles in our Catholic faith, giving us a taste of this dimension of "sign" in our bodies. This is an intuition we have largely lost in our modern world — to see the physical realm as a symbol of deep, spiritual truth — so let's rediscover that heritage through the Church and begin to apply it to our menstrual cycles. This first mode of inquiry will have us start with God, work our way through symbols, and then see how these insights apply to our cycles. In my mind, I visualize this as a sort of top-down form of meditation.

> *If we fail to recognize God's image living in our very bodies, then we will be hard-pressed to understand or appreciate any of the other roles we play in life, even those beautiful vocational roles of wife, religious sister, or consecrated virgin.*

After that, we will embark on a second mode of inquiry that will go in the other direction: We will begin by observing the natural function and design of our bodies and then contemplate what that may symbolize about ourselves in relationship to one another and God. This is more like a bottom-up approach. By using both of these modes, we will be able to meditate more fully on how women *image* and *are like* God through the biological function of our menstrual cycles.

I should conclude this chapter by acknowledging that what we do here with menstrual cycles could be done with other body systems and functions as well. It would be misleading to suggest that the things we reflect on here will be an exhaustive look at the way the female body images God. This is merely one small element of the way our female bodies "speak" the language of sign, but I believe it is a particularly important one because it is so central to the lived experience of female embodiment as distinct from male embodiment. Women are so often ashamed or embarrassed by this unique function of our bodies: If we can learn to see the divine symbolism behind our cycles — not for their valuable function in reproduction, but in and of themselves — how can that help us embrace and live out our *imago Dei* more fully?

CHAPTER 4

The *Imago Dei* in the Paradox of the Circle

To begin our reflection on women's cycles in the *imago Dei,* we can first look at the rich symbolism that is already present in our Catholic faith. The Church, following the traditions of Judaism, has always utilized tangible symbols to communicate specific ideas, creating a rich visual language for us to meditate on particular spiritual realities. For example: A painting of a saint holding a palm branch calls us to contemplate the victory she won over death through martyrdom. If the saint is holding a lily, we should understand that to mean that he was considered pure and chaste. These are examples of specific objects, but this language of symbolism also carries through in the use of basic shapes. For example, a triangle will typically refer to the Trinity. A star can represent the historical star of Bethlehem, but it can also represent the general idea that we should actively be seeking knowledge of goodness and truth. Drawing on this rich inheritance, we can start our meditation by the way we visualize, or symbolically represent, the "shape" that a menstrual cycle takes — that of a circle. Is there a way in which the embodied *circle* of events within a woman's body actually images God?

When we think about where circles appear in our faith, we might immediately think of a halo around the head of an angel or saint, which is meant to indicate their holiness. But why was a circle chosen to represent this? We may take it for granted that a halo *is* a circular shape, but there are actually many different styles of halo used in sacred art, including almond-shaped haloes (also called mandorla), triangular haloes (typically reserved for persons of the Trinity), and even square haloes. This last one is worth focusing on, because a square halo is used to indicate someone who is still living: usually a donor who would commission the work, or someone like an abbot or pope — so as to distinguish them from the saints depicted. So circular haloes are not just used to represent holiness; specifically, they represent holiness as it is expressed in a glorified state in heaven. A living, earthbound person gets a square, whereas a holy person in heaven gets a circle.

This distinction gives us some insight into how circles were viewed by our ancient and medieval forebears, who are primarily responsible for the symbolic tradition we have inherited. What did *they* think was important and different about the circle as compared with other shapes? Among other things, the circle was understood to be a perfect shape, fitting for the spheres of heaven; whereas even a square — with sides of equal length and perfect right angles — belongs more fittingly to the sort of created perfection found on earth. From that observation, we can dive into a few of the specific ways in which circles are used in the Church to express aspects of God, and think about how our own menstrual cycles might image those aspects as well.

GOD WITHOUT BEGINNING

When we look at a circle, how do we know where the beginning is? A well-trained eye may be able to look at a circle drawn by hand and discern the slightest dot where the artist seems to have first put pen to paper; but this would obviously be an imperfect circle, drawn by human hands. When we imagine a perfect circle, however, we see that there is no obvious spot where the shape must be said to begin. Perhaps this could be said of other shapes as well, but all of the other regular shapes are polygons, meaning they have straight sides with edges and corners, one of which could easily be identified as a starting point. Not to belabor the idea too much, but even though one could, in theory, begin drawing a triangle in the middle of one of its sides, we will almost always begin drawing the shape at one of the points.

When a circle is used in our faith, it communicates this idea of *eternity,* being without beginning or end. As I sit here at my desk, it is December, and I can see the shape of my Advent wreath on the coffee table. The candles represent Christ, the Light of the World, who has entered time by assuming human nature. Yet the underlying shape of the circular wreath represents his eternal, divine nature, which is completely outside of time and has no beginning. As the psalmist sings:

> Lord, you have been our dwelling place
> in all generations.
> Before the mountains were brought forth,
> or ever you had formed the earth and the world,
> from everlasting to everlasting you are God. (Psalm 90:1–2)

We cannot pinpoint a beginning or starting point with God, just as we cannot find one single point which is the beginning of the circle.

Saint Thomas writes about this when he describes how there are actually five natural "proofs" of God's existence, the first three of which essentially boil down to the observation that there has to be something that is not moved, or caused, or contingent upon something else. In other words, there has to be something that does not have a beginning: "And this everyone understands to be God (I. Q. 2, art. 2)."[1]

So how might this relate to our menstrual cycles? Doesn't our period clearly mark the beginning of a new cycle?

The answer, simply put, is both yes and no. We have decided as a matter of convention that our period bleeds will serve as the line of demarcation between different cycles, because it's useful to mark the start of a cycle with a biological event that all women can observe. But even among Natural Family Planning methods, there are further nuances that are not universally agreed upon. For the method that I teach, we will define the first day of a new cycle as the day bleeding reaches a flow, not just spotting, before midnight. Not all methods make this same distinction — or, if they do, they only make it if there are three or more days of spotting prior to the start of flow. Still other methods will have different conventions based on whether their biomarker tracking is tied to a particular device that gives instruction on an alternate way to count days. All this is to say that a convention as seemingly simple as using bleeding days to mark the beginning of a new cycle is actually not all that simple. And so the most important thing when you are tracking your own cycle or following a particular method is to be internally consistent: always use the same criteria to determine which day to count as the start of a new cycle.

In other words, when we are talking about menstrual cycles, we rely heavily on conventions that are meaningful and useful for us as humans, rather than articulating some deep, metaphysical reality about cycles themselves. There is nothing that necessitates using bleeding days as our determining factor for the start of a new cycle. We could just as meaningfully identify ovulation as the beginning of a new cycle. Or we could choose to begin with the proliferation of endometrial lining in the uterus, as I did in the story of the kingdom in our first chapter. Unlike some other biological processes such as pregnancy, a woman's menstrual cycle has no single event that needs to be called "the beginning."

To drive the point home further, remember what we discussed earlier: Our tidy narrative of a new cycle beginning at a bleed is not quite the full truth, either. The egg that is released at ovulation following a bleed didn't simply begin maturing roughly two weeks prior, when hormones reset during the period. The egg that will be released during that cycle has actually been developing for about ninety days already, meaning that it has undergone many waves of hormonal surges over the past few cycles to help it reach its current state. From the egg's perspective, a single cycle is actually a series of many cycles: One circle is composed of many, but their multitude is concealed by the single, simple shape.

Perhaps, then, we could think about *menarche* as the beginning of this entire cyclical sequence. This is when a girl gets her first bleed and begins the long process of hormone pathway regulation, which will eventually lead to regular menstrual cycles. Wouldn't that be a clear beginning? To that I will have to answer again, yes and no! While it is true that a girl will have a first bleed, this event may or may not actually be a true period. We have already discussed how ovulation is the main event in a cycle and that a bleed that is preceded by ovulation is a period; but it is also possible to have anovulatory bleeds that were not preceded by ovulation and are caused by a different sort of hormonal event. So a bleed definitely indicates that a girl's body is somewhere in the process of this menstrual cycle; but a bleed alone — even a first bleed — isn't as clear-cut as it may seem.

Of course, we must admit that yes, there *is* a beginning to a woman's cycle, even if we aren't able to pinpoint exactly when that is. Anything related to the human body cannot actually be without a beginning, since it is created, and so this particular aspect of the circle symbolism is quite limited. But the other half of the eternity symbolism is that eternity is not just without beginning — it is without end. And it is possible to speak about finite things, like our bodies, being "without end."

GOD WITHOUT END

If we revisit the symbolism of the Advent wreath, we can add another layer of interpretation to the circle, which directly relates to the coming of Christ: Through the Son, God is now inviting us back to the opportunity to share eternal life with him. We have already discussed how Adam and Eve's transgression in the Garden of Eden negatively impacted their connection to God. But through Jesus Christ, the path opens again for us to be restored in that original unity and justice. This is why a traditional Advent wreath is made of evergreen sprigs — because the circle reminds us of the promise of everlasting life.

This concept of everlasting life, or existence without end, properly belongs to God in his divine nature. Paul writes, "To the King of ages, immortal, invisible, the only God, be honor and glory for ever and ever. Amen" (1 Tm 1:17). God, as the cause of his own existence, can never cease to be. He can never cause himself out of existence: The Divine nature has what we might call a *necessary* existence. God exists because he is Being, and Being what he is, he cannot cease to be. You can even hear a circularity in that explanation!

The joy of Christianity is to proclaim that despite having a beginning, it is not a foregone conclusion that all creatures must likewise have an end. In fact, Jesus himself tells us that this is not so. In Matthew's Gospel, he speaks about the final judgment. Those who have turned their back on him by neglecting service to others "will go away into eternal punishment, but the righteous into eternal life" (Mt 25:46). We sometimes miss the fact that in both of these cases, our existence continues *for eternity.* The key difference is that some are admitted to eternal *life,* which is the opposite of separation from God. Thus, "life" is not just about existence. It is directly equated to a union with God and is supported in the writings of many saints. For example, quoting St. Cyril of Jerusalem, the *Catechism* states: "True and subsistent life consists in this: the Father, through the Son and in the Holy Spirit, pouring out his heavenly gifts on all things without exception. Thanks to his mercy, we too, men that we are, have received the inalienable promise of eternal life" (1050).

> *The joy of Christianity is to proclaim that despite having a beginning, it is not a foregone conclusion that all creatures must likewise have an end.*

How does all this relate to the symbolism of the circle? We know that women go through menopause — the cessation of menstrual cycles — and so it cannot be said that once our cycles begin, they proceed for eternity. But remember what we have said before: Our bodies, as part of the physical universe, have a sacramental quality — pointing us toward divine or invisible realities through this concept of "sign." So, when we think about the circle as a visual representation of our physical menstrual cycles, we need not think that every aspect of the comparison needs to be exact. Instead, we can look at the general concepts that are signified: specifically, how the female reproductive system is an embodiment of cyclicality, which, among other things, symbolizes the eternity of God.

Let me interject a word of caution and clarification about

everything we will say in the following chapters: When we try to assign particular aspects of God either to the female or male body exclusively, I fear that we risk missing the whole point entirely. What I mean is that in Genesis we are told that male and female are *both* images of God. So, while it is true that we learn certain things about God through meditating on the image of woman, and we learn certain things about God through meditating on the image of man, we learn even more about God when we also meditate on the complementary union of man and woman, together. So if I suggest that a woman's reproductive system images the eternal life of God, it is not meant to be reductive and suggest that *only* a woman's reproductive system does this. Instead, hopefully this can serve as a model for how we could also approach the question of a man's reproductive system imaging God in its own unique way, and how both male and female image the eternal life of God together.

EXITUS — REDITUS

As Christians we believe that all things come from God. St. John the Evangelist tells us that "all things were made through him" (Jn 1:3), a creative emanation that is often called *exitus.* As creatures, our mere existence is an *exitus*: a coming forth from God, who is the source of all being. Yet we are not called to simply "go forth" from God; we are also called to *return* to him. St. Thomas Aquinas reminds us that "God is the last end of man" (*Summa Theologiae*, I-II, Q1, art.8), meaning that union with God is the purpose of our existence. So if we begin life with an *exitus,* then there must be a *reditus,* a returning — or reuniting — with God.

A true *reditus* for any human action will not be passive. If we think about how we return to God in general, we'd be speaking of the cultivation of virtue and the pursuit of holiness. We can only return to God and be wholly reunited with him when our wills desire God alone. And because we have free will, we know that this union with God must be actively chosen and demonstrated through love. So how does this relate to our cycles?

We can picture the movement of this "emanation" and "return" as a sort of circle that actually does have a beginning and an end, both of which are exactly the same — namely, God. As we meditate on these concepts, we have a particularly apt way of thinking about the uterine cycle of women. We have already seen that the menstrual cycle is a very complicated symphony between hormones working in both the ovaries and the uterus. When we choose to focus on the development of the egg, we are particularly focusing on what might be called the *ovarian* cycle, because the events take place in the ovaries. However, the uterine cycle is primarily a story about the building up of endometrial lining, that nutrient-rich layer that would support a baby in the initial stages of pregnancy, but which is shed during a woman's period in the absence of pregnancy.

We can picture the movement of this "emanation" and "return" as a sort of circle that actually does have a beginning and an end, both of which are exactly the same — namely, God.

This shedding of lining reminds us of an *exitus,* a coming forth of life from its source. Of course, the more perfect analogy here would be giving birth, but regardless of her pregnancy status, a woman's body will "birth" the contents of her womb when the ovulatory cycle is complete. Yet our period blood does not return to our bodies to be reused, so what is the corresponding *reditus?*

Perhaps our *reditus,* in relationship to the uterine cycle, could be seen as the generous choice our bodies often make to return to the laborious task of building up more uterine lining and going through the cycle again. Unless there exists some other health impediment, a woman's body will go right back to expending nutrients, releasing hormones, and starting the process over. Admittedly, this isn't an aspect of our biological function that is completely under our control. We don't use our free will to "activate" a new cycle each time, but it's also not the case that we are completely passive, either. Women do need to choose to steward our bodies in order to keep them well-nourished and equipped to perform the task of a menstrual cycle. Practically speaking, this means supplying our bodies with iron, which is lost through our periods, eating healthy amounts of fat and protein, managing external stressors that are under our control, and so much more. We will speak later in this book about some specific care that our bodies need throughout the cycle, but for now the point is that this *reditus,* or the *return* of life-giving nourishment to fuel another cycle, is something that does require an element of choice. This doesn't mean that every woman is somehow morally obligated to "optimize" her cycles through some complicated diet, exercise, or mental health program. But, at a minimum, we do need to give our bodies the basic care they need to support our cycles, or risk losing them altogether.[2]

What I love about this *exitus-reditus* imagery is that it keeps us from imagining that our cycles need to be "perfect circles" in order to symbolize all of the things we are speaking of here. Most women are not going to have perfectly balanced cycles in the sense that our follicular phases and luteal phases are exactly the same length from month to month. That's an illustration we can use in a textbook to conceptualize the idea of cycle phases and relative lengths, but most women will have a lot more variation in their cycles than that. This is especially true of my clients who have irregular cycles, whether that's due to an underlying condition like polycystic ovary syndrome or something else.

By envisioning the symbolism of the circle as an emanation and return, we allow ourselves the freedom to picture our cycles less like a perfect circle and more like the flight path of a boomerang, which can have wildly different trajectories based on wind patterns, how hard the object is thrown, angle of entry, and so much else! So, too, are the varying cycles of women, some of which may seem to have a perfectly even pattern like a circle — and others that may seem to veer one way or another for a while, but which eventually return to their source and begin again.

Perhaps it may seem like the theme of *exitus* and *reditus* is not really a way in which we image God, because it is so tied to our creaturehood. The Father does not proceed from and return to himself. But listen to the words of Christ, as he addresses his disciples prior to his arrest in the Gospel According to John: "I came from the Father and have come into the world; again, I am leaving the world and going back to the Father" (16:28). The Son of God shows us that the life of the Trinity, wrapped up in the mystery of the Incarnation, is one in which even the Divine Persons emanate from and return to one another. Therefore, through Christ, we can also say that the theme of *exitus* and *reditus*, which is specifically embodied through women's cycles, can be a part of how we *image* God.

A circle is thus a fitting entry into this discussion of image, for in the abstract symbol of the circle we see how the Church expresses God's eternal life without beginning or end. We see that the circle also represents our own journey from and back toward God, perfectly demonstrated by Christ himself. By delving into this rich symbolism already present in the Church's theology, we can see that our menstrual cycles share many of the qualities of the circle — imaging through an embodied, very concrete symbolism, these wonderful aspects of God.

CHAPTER 5

The *Imago Dei* in the Liturgy of the Church

Growing up, I heard a story about how one of my aunts was tempted to walk out of a wedding at which Ephesians 5 was proclaimed. I don't know any of the details, because I heard it as a kid and none of the important grown-up information registered at the time. All I internalized is that Ephesians 5 makes some women angry, and is a portion of the Bible that should be just skimmed over because it doesn't really apply to today's modern world. I am glad that my understanding of Scripture has matured since then, but we still have to admit that this reading can certainly be a challenge:

> Be subject to one another out of reverence for Christ. Wives, be subject to your husbands, as to the Lord. For

the husband is the head of the wife as Christ is the head of the Church, his body, and is himself its Savior. As the Church is subject to Christ, so let wives also be subject in everything to their husbands. Husbands, love your wives, as Christ loved the Church and gave himself up for her, that he might sanctify her, having cleansed her by the washing of water with the word, that he might present the Church to himself in splendor, without spot or wrinkle or any such thing, that she might be holy and without blemish. Even so husbands should love their wives as their own bodies. He who loves his wife loves himself. For no man ever hates his own flesh, but nourishes and cherishes it, as Christ does the Church, because we are members of his body. "For this reason a man shall leave his father and mother and be joined to his wife, and the two shall become one flesh." This is a great mystery, and I mean in reference to Christ and the Church; however, let each one of you love his wife as himself, and let the wife see that she respects her husband (vv. 21–33).

Ladies, whether you adore Ephesians 5 or whether you abhor it because you've never heard it preached in a way that feels respectful to your womanhood, the fact remains that this particular passage drops an incredible bomb on every Christian conversation about marriage, the Second Coming of Christ, and even Christology itself. Here's the most important line: "This is a great mystery, and I mean in reference to Christ and the Church."

THE CHURCH AS THE BODY OF CHRIST
What, precisely, is Saint Paul applying to Christ and the Church? First, let us be clear that by "Church" we do not mean "the building where worship takes place," but rather the composite iden-

tity of those who are baptized in Christ. Saint Paul says that the Church is the union of those who are "all baptized into one body" (1 Cor 12:13). It is precisely this entity to which he applies the words of Genesis: "For this reason a man will leave his father and mother and be joined to his wife, and the two will become one flesh." The man is Christ, and the Church is his bride.

Before we return to meditation on our menstrual cycles, let's sit with this image of Christ, the Divine Son. Though he did not cease to be with the Father and the Holy Spirit, he "emptied himself, taking the form of a servant, being born in the likeness of men" (Phil 2:7). In a sense, the Son left his home to be joined to his wife — the Church — so that we could become one flesh with him. Even now, our Divine Bridegroom calls us to his heavenly home, to the final consummation of God's marriage to his people. We, as members of the Body of Christ, which is the Church, are called to be *one flesh* with our Creator.

> *We, as members of the Body of Christ, which is the Church, are called to be* one flesh *with our Creator.*

When I think about this, it makes me wonder how our male counterparts resonate with the fleshy aspect of wedding imagery in Scripture and in Tradition. Does the idea of becoming a "bride of Christ" through the Church make them a little squeamish? As a sort of baseline test, I think we'd all admit that a sixteen-year-old girl with religious inclinations would probably be a lot more comfortable thinking about being a "bride of Christ" than would her male counterpart. Here is our parallel, as women, to the difficulty we expressed earlier: Jesus Christ has a physically male body, and this means that Christ is not with women in exactly the same way he is with men. Could we conversely say that because Jesus' bride is the Church, he is with women in a particular way that he is not with men? This is a very careful way of suggesting that Christ possesses two bodies: One of them is biologically and physically male. The other body, joined with him as one flesh, is the body of his bride — the Church. And this second body lives an incredibly cyclical life, through her rich rhythm of liturgical prayer.

WHAT IS LITURGY?

In general, Catholics speak about two different categories of prayer, both of which are deeply important: liturgical prayer and devotional prayer. Within these categories are various forms and expressions of prayer, which are outlined beautifully in the final section of the *Catechism of the Catholic Church*: Our Church has handed down rich writing and tradition about prayer, because prayer is nothing less than each person's "vital and personal relationship with the living and true God" (2558).[1] Here, we'll focus on prayer as liturgy, rather than prayer as devotion.

In *Sacrosanctum Concilium*, the liturgical constitution approved during the Second Vatican Council, we read:

> Rightly, then, the liturgy is considered as an exercise of the priestly office of Jesus Christ. ... In the liturgy the whole public worship is performed by the Mystical Body of Jesus Christ, that is, by the Head and His members.
>
> From this it follows that every liturgical celebration, because it is an action of Christ the priest and of His Body which is the Church, is a sacred action surpassing all others; no other action of the Church can equal its efficacy by the same title and to the same degree.[2]

To sum up a very complicated discussion that has spanned the life of the Church, liturgy (*leitourgia* in the Greek) can be defined as the public work done by members of the Body of Christ, in union with the priestly power of Jesus Christ, for the redemption of the entire Church. Devotional prayer has a more private nature — whether done by an individual or a group, devotion is not so much about the official work of the redemption of the Church, but about advancing in personal holiness.

Devotional prayer can be exercised by any person seeking a relationship with God, unlike liturgy, which can only be done by a baptized person. This is because when we are baptized, each individual Christian is given the power to participate in Christ's threefold role as priest, prophet, and king. The *Catechism* explicitly states: "Jesus Christ is the one whom the Father anointed with the Holy Spirit and established as priest, prophet, and king. The whole People of God participates in these three offices of Christ and bears the responsibilities for mission and service that flow from them" (783). Whereas the Jewish people relied on priests to offer all of the sacrifices on behalf of the people, Christians are able to exercise the priestly role of Christ by directly offering sacrifices for themselves and others. This is not the same thing as saying that all of the baptized are able to receive holy orders — women's ordination is a closed issue within the Church. What it does mean is that women and men are both called to participate in the work of redemption through the Body of Christ, which is the Church. When we engage in this official work, we are offering the highest prayer we can, because we are explicitly participating in Christ's own work.

Liturgical prayer can therefore be thought of as the official work of the Church on behalf of her Bridegroom. And what is that work? Perhaps we are most familiar with the Mass as a form of liturgy, but we can break that down further. Within the Mass, there are actually two distinct, but related, liturgies. The first is the Liturgy of the Word, through which the faithful encounter and consume the Word revealed through Sacred Scripture. The second is the Liturgy of the Eucharist, through which the faithful encounter and consume the Word, incarnate in the person of

Jesus Christ, under the appearances of bread and wine.

The other liturgical prayer of the Church is the Divine Office, also known as the Liturgy of the Hours, which sanctifies the day through the recitation of specific prayers at various "hours," spaced at roughly three-hour intervals throughout the day. The psalms are the organizing principle of the Divine Office; they are spread throughout a four-week rotation.

THE CYCLICAL LIFE OF LITURGY

The life of the Church — the Bride of Christ, who is also mysteriously the Body of Christ — is expressed through her cyclicality, much like biological women whose menstrual cycles impact so much of our physical, emotional, and even spiritual lives. When we observe the liturgical life of the Church, we see how layered this cyclical life is.

First, we can think about an individual Mass. During Mass, the members of the parish — your local incarnation of the Church — gather together in the church building. We do so in order to exercise our priestly office by participating in the holy sacrifice of the Mass, but we also come in order to receive the abundant graces offered through reception of the Eucharist. We could have called this supreme act of worship the "Divine Liturgy" as our Eastern Catholic and other Christian brethren do, but Catholics use this strange word "Mass," which comes from the Latin phrase: *Ite, missa est.* In English we could translate that literally to mean "Go! It is the dismissal." But to capture the meaning, a better phrase might actually be "Go! You are commissioned!" In other words, we go to Mass in order to make an offering of ourselves to God and to receive him in the great Sacrament of the Eucharist, but the purpose of this sacred memorial is to strengthen us for the great mission.

Here, again, we encounter this concept of cyclicality as *exitus* and *reditus* — emanation and return. The Mass gathers us from our various individual lives, so we can be strengthened together and sent out yet again. That is the first layer of liturgical cyclicality in the Church, which is expressed in both the physical movements of the people of God coming and going, as well as in the spiritual movements of all who offer themselves, receive the Lord, and are commissioned to go out and offer the Lord to others through themselves … only to return and do it all again at the next Mass.

If we focus on the fact that Sunday is the day of obligation when all the faithful are required to attend Mass, we could say that this liturgical act happens on a weekly cycle; however, as members of the Church who have received holy orders, priests are obligated to celebrate Mass every day. Thus we can think about Mass as the *circadian* cycle of the Church's liturgical life.

The next layer of cyclicality is found in the rhythm of prayer prescribed by the Liturgy of the Hours. This prayer is currently structured in a four-week rotation of psalms and readings called the "Ordinary." In order to know which prayers should be said that day, you need to know which day of the week it is and which week of the rotation you are in. For example, the day I am writing happens to be Friday of Week I in the Divine Office. In a couple of days, it will be Sunday of Week II. The psalms and readings will be specific to that day. Once you've been through all of Week I, II, III, and IV, then you start back over with Sunday of Week I and the rotation begins again.

Of all the different layers of cyclicality we can reflect on in the liturgy, this four-week psalter matches most closely with the biological length of a woman's menstrual cycle, which is known as an *infradian* cycle. We will come back to this in a later chapter when we discuss Mary, but four weeks roughly corresponds to the lunar cycle, which is the basis of months within our annual calendar. Here, we can think about the deep connection between our spirits and our bodies: It seems that our souls naturally incline to rhythms of prayer that correspond to the rhythms of biological, embodied life.

I often like to quote a line from the US bishops' quick informational flier on gestures at Mass. The document says, "We are creatures of body as well as spirit, so our prayer is not confined to our minds and hearts. It is expressed by our bodies as well. When our bodies are engaged in our prayer, we pray with our whole person. Using our entire being in prayer helps us to pray with greater attentiveness."[3] While this speaks specifically to the importance of engaging our bodies in prayer, it also hints at something that our ancestors in faith were much more attuned to than we moderns tend to be: The body is itself a locus of prayer. Therefore, our bodily experiences of time-keeping through the celestial events of days, months, and years are elements that should be brought to prayer so that we might pray as "whole persons." This is not a new idea: Liturgy expert Martin Connell explains that especially in the early days of the Church, there was a marked connection between "creed (what the Church believed) and chronometry (how the Church kept or measured time)."[4] Thus the rising and falling of the sun, the waxing and waning of the moon, and the passing of the seasons throughout the year are not just about marking time. They are physical, finite manifestations of God's eternal action in the world that we — as embodied souls — are invited to participate in, again and again.

On top of the circadian cycle of Mass and the infradian cycle of the Liturgy of the Hours, the liturgical calendar builds out another layer of cyclicality in the Church's life: an annual cycle. The liturgical calendar contains feasts, which happen on specific days and may commemorate a particular saint (e.g., Saint Margaret of Scotland), teaching (e.g., the Immaculate Conception of the Blessed Virgin Mary), significant ecclesiastical event (e.g., the dedication of St. John Lateran cathedral), or seasons (Advent, Christmas, Ordinary Time, Lent, and Easter).

We can see wisdom in the way the Church asks us to pace ourselves and experience different aspects of our faith through the liturgical year. Specifically, we have times when we are asked to pause, reflect, and slow down. The penitential seasons of Advent and Lent are meant to prepare us for the feasts of Christmas and Easter, but they are not only preparatory; in and of themselves they help form and deepen our collective and individual prayer lives. These seasons may be understood as akin to the luteal phase in the menstrual cycle, when women's bodies are actively preparing for a pregnancy or period, or even perhaps the days of menses when the old layers of endometrial lining are shed in order to make room for new growth. Festive liturgical seasons like Christmas and Easter may be likened to the ovulatory days in a woman's cycle, when her body is primed for connection, activity, and the expenditure of valuable energy. Thus we see the Church and the biology of a woman's body reflecting the wisdom of the Book of Ecclesiastes: "For everything there is a season, and a time for every matter under heaven" (3:1).

On top of the circadian, infradian, and annual cycles of the Church, we also have a three-year cycle of readings for the Mass, known as the lectionary. When we think about the life of the Church we can see that the Bride of Christ — the Body of Christ — experiences cycles upon cycles upon cycles. In my talks with young adult groups, I put forward the idea that our Church is like a *super*woman: Her Body experiences a cyclicality that extends far beyond what women biologically experience in our bodies. It seems sometimes as if God looked at his image in woman, saw that it was very good, and then said, "I'm going to make my Bride just like that … but *more.*" Or to put it perhaps another way that is more fitting for our understanding of God: "Let us make woman in Our image. She will be a type of Our beloved Bride, with a rich cyclical life to guide her."

WHAT ABOUT MEN?

Let's pause to ponder the role of men in the life of the Church, especially since men are capable of embodying a different sort of priesthood than women. When we think of the Church as feminine and of having this cyclical life, what does that mean for the men who are equally members of her Body?

This is one of my favorite things to ponder, because it makes me appreciate how God has designed the world and his plan of salvation to work. In the beginning, he made male and female, both equally his images, expressing aspects of his Divine Nature in different ways as individuals and communally as a pair. Through Christ, true God and true man, God ushered in a new sacramental life in the Church.

And thus, by baptism, Eucharist and confirmation — the sacraments of initiation — biological men actually become, by grace and participation, what women are internally by nature: cyclical beings.

Note the distinction that is made: men and women — along with most creatures here on earth — equally experience the sort of cyclicality that is imposed through the daily rhythms of the sun and the monthly rhythms of the moon. This is an external cyclicality to which we are subject, given to us by timekeeping movements and heavenly bodies that are outside of ourselves. It is not the same sort of cyclicality experienced in the life of the Church, which comes internally from her own creativity and work. To understand the importance of this distinction, we can look at the axiom, articulated by Thomas Aquinas, that in all things "grace perfects nature" (see *ST*, I.1.8, reply to Obj. 2). Following the example of many great thinkers in the Church, such as Augustine and the Venerable Bede, it is important to say that our liturgical year is not independent of the seasons or the passing of celestial bodies. But we should also say that the liturgical year takes the foundation of the natural passing of time, and elevates it to its full potential, which is the union of created time with the eternal life of God. And the Church is the only entity that can accomplish that task.

In other words, men and women are naturally both subject to the passing of time as dictated by the sun and moon. But through participation in the priestly identity of Christ, men and women are no longer merely subject to time: Instead, we become creators and keepers of an entirely new dimension of time in the liturgical life of the Church. Without people on this planet, there would still be days and nights and years. But there would not be Advent. Or Easter. Or even Ordinary Time. Just like various hormones, organs, and systems are required to create the intricate work of a menstrual cycle in a woman's body, the various members of the Church — through liturgy — are all required to make these layers of cyclicality happen in the Body of Christ.

LITURGY IN THE NEW JERUSALEM

Now we can bring forward an aspect of cyclicality that we haven't yet touched upon: the fact that women don't have cycles for our entire lives. Rather, there are specific times when our cycles begin (menarche) and when they stop (menopause). We stated in the introductory chapters that human women are one of the very few species we know of that actually go through menopause, which prompts us to pause and consider whether that has any significance for us as creatures.

Let's go back to this key concept that "woman" signifies the Body of Christ, which is the Church. Is there a way that the beginning and the end of women's menstrual cycles are signified or lived out also in the life of the Church, specifically in the context of liturgy? For women, there are three major "phases" that we go through in life, each marked by a key transitional event. First, we go through the phase of life when we are girls who do not yet have cycles. Once we get our first bleed, we enter the second phase of our lives, which is called the "reproductive years," meaning our cycles are present and we could potentially bring life into the world. This phase ends at menopause, which ushers in the third phase of post-menopausal life.

By analogy, we could perhaps say that the liturgical life of the Church, as we know it right now, is like the reproductive years in a woman's life, when she experiences her menstrual cycle. Through the sacraments, she is able to bring a new sort of life into the world. We see how the baptismal font functions like a womb in Jesus' conversation with Nicodemus: "Jesus answered him, 'Truly, truly, I say to you, unless one is born anew, he cannot see the kingdom of God.' Nicodemus said to him, 'How can a man be born when he is old? Can he enter a second time into his mother's womb and be born?' Jesus answered, 'Truly, truly, I say to you, unless one is born of water and the Spirit, he cannot enter the kingdom of God'" (Jn 3:3–5).

While obviously not a perfect analogy, we could consider that Jesus' death on the cross — the spilling of Divine Blood — is the key event that marks the introduction of the Church's existence and her sacramental life. Continuing in the Gospel of John, this imagery is made very clear: "But one of the soldiers pierced [Jesus'] side with a spear, and at once there came out blood and water" (19:34). Aquinas explains in his commentary on John that "it is these two things which are especially associated with two sacraments: water with the sacrament of baptism, and blood with the Eucharist ... this event was also prefigured, for just as from the side of Christ, sleeping on the cross, there flowed blood and water, which makes the Church holy, so from the side of the sleeping Adam there was formed the woman, who prefigured the Church."[5]

So, did the Church have a phase of life before her "reproductive years"? One might say that, like Eve, the Church simply came into existence out of nothing except the body of her groom. Yet, we also know that the Church — composed of both Gentiles and

Jews — was preceded in history by God's chosen people, Israel. This nation was already called God's "beloved," and the Old Testament is sprinkled with imagery of Israel as the lover, as the wife of the Lord. So perhaps we can meditate on the way God betrothed himself to his bride while she was yet immature and had not yet attained the fruitfulness of her sacramental life. Then, after the coming of the Bridegroom, the Church entered into a new phase of her identity through the liturgical and sacramental life. So we can see that perhaps there are two out of three phases of life represented here. Is there a third — one that can mirror post-menopausal life?

Speaking purely from the perspective of history, we know that we have not yet reached the fullness of time, when all things will be brought together in Christ. In the Book of Revelation, John sees "a new heaven and a new earth; for the first heaven and the first earth had passed away, and the sea was no more. And I saw the holy city, new Jerusalem, coming down out of heaven from God, prepared as a bride adorned for her husband" (21:1–2). At the end of time, the Church will be revealed in her true identity as the New Jerusalem — as she passes into yet another phase of her life, beyond those reproductive years, into a sort of menopause.

Does this mean that in this new existence, the cyclical rhythm of liturgy will cease? Similarly to how a woman's body goes through menopause, will there be a cessation of liturgical cycles? Here again, our analogy is not quite perfect, but it can be a way in which we ponder the symbolism found in menopause that women go through. If we strip the concept of liturgy down to its most basic component of worship and praise of God, then we have to assert that this form of liturgy will never cease. The book of Revelation is full of multitudes, singing praise over and over again to the Lord before the throne. That will never cease, because, really, that is the fulfillment of our human nature — the ability to stand face to face with God and to worship him in spirit and truth for all eternity.

Yet in another sense, we can and should say that the cyclical liturgical life of the Church will be transfigured in this New Jerusalem and will cease to be what it was before. All of our liturgy right now is simultaneously looking forward and looking back. The act of *anamnesis,* the "un-forgetting" of God's saving acts, permeates all of our worship but most especially the Mass, as we re-present Christ's ultimate sacrifice on the cross. Yet liturgy is also an expression of the hope that longs for the future consummation of all things in Christ. We see this perfectly in the season of Advent, which not only helps us to remember the birth of Christ, but to look forward to his second coming. After that fulfillment, we do not yet know what form our worship will take.

Drawing together all the images we have explored, we can posit that the way in which a woman goes through life is itself a sort of *image* of the life of the Church. She begins as a young girl, which is like God calling the nation of Israel to himself, as an entity that has not yet actualized her potential in the womb of her baptismal font. Then, she enters menarche — the first shedding of blood — and goes through puberty to become a woman, living cyclically through her reproductive years, which is like the current liturgical life of the Church. Finally, she undergoes another transition that by no means negates her womanhood, but transforms it to femininity beyond cycles, which is like the Church transformed into the fullness of the New Jerusalem at the wedding feast of the Lamb.

CHAPTER 6

The *Imago Dei* in Superabundant Generosity

I am going to admit something in this book what I have previously admitted to exactly three people, because not only is it a bit embarrassing, but it's also weirdly niche. Are you ready?

Not all that long ago, I had to turn down an offer to hang out with a Dominican friar at a pub because of a heavy period bleed. I bled not only through my super maxi pad; I had also overflowed and filled my period underwear and soaked through a pair of pants. This is after having used up my arsenal of pads during the previous five hours. Fortunately, I was prepared with a very black ensemble and nobody was aware that I was undergoing the menstrual equivalent of Mount Vesuvius. But there was no way I was going to sit down on a bar stool for another hour. It was time to go home.

Hopefully, anyone reading this strange confession is able to recognize that I was in dire need of medical attention at this point — which I did eventually get, by the way. Yet despite the fact that this was an abnormal and unhealthy amount of bleeding, I experienced an oddly calm sense of respect for the fact that my body was able to produce so much endometrial lining during a relatively short amount of time.

I remember an off-handed, snide remark high school boys would pass around: you should never trust anything that can bleed for seven days without dying. Of course they were referring to menstruation and casting it in a very negative light, but behind the insult is the acknowledgment that menstruation is a strange and powerful force. And the occurrence of a menstrual bleed is something that serves as a fundamental experiential divide between the sexes.

In this chapter, we're going to ponder our menstrual cycles under one of the key aspects Pope St. John Paul II highlights about the feminine genius: generosity. In his 1995 *Letter to Women*, John Paul II twice mentions the way in which women are particularly generous in serving and offering themselves up for the good of others. He says that this generosity is expressed in the "heart of the family" and areas of education and care "extending well beyond the family: nurseries, schools, universities, social service agencies, parishes, associations and movements" (*Letter to Women*, 9). Particularly, we'll contemplate how our menstrual cycles can help us better understand the superabundant generosity and care that God extends to all of creation.

SUPERABUNDANCE IN ATTENTION AND CARE

Putting aside the obvious medical issues I was experiencing in the previous story, our periods are the visible, external sign of an incredible amount of work that is done by our bodies throughout the menstrual cycle. Even a small amount of period flow is the product of a rich network of blood vessels and uterine cells that have been meticulously designed and curated by a symphony of hormones over the course of many weeks.

A few years ago, I was deep in the work of creating my Cycle Prep program to teach girls about menarche. I had been so careful in crafting the language of that program, focusing on making sure that I had given the girls positive scripts about the good, hard work their body was doing to produce this cycle. I wanted them to develop a healthy respect for the function of their female reproductive system, so that even if they felt anxious or grossed out or otherwise awful about their periods, they would at least know that with a period, their body was doing exactly what it was designed to do.

I had not prepared for the fact that I needed to tell myself that same thing. I wasn't aware of all of the negative comments I routinely thought to myself as I cared for my body during a period, or as I experienced various changes throughout my cycle. But one day, I surprised myself by becoming my own case study. It was a heavy day of bleeding, and previously I would have rolled my eyes and made some snide remark to myself about this "bloody mess" while I cleaned up. However, after spending all of that effort composing positive scripts for girls, my immediate reaction this time was something different: I saw the amount of blood I had lost, and my immediate thought was, "Wow. That's impressive. Way to go, uterus."

Through building up these positive scripts, I had been given the eyes to see my period in a completely new and positive light. And this led to another series of personal reflections that ended up being incorporated into the Cycle Prep program: namely, that our bodies are ridiculously generous in providing new endometrial lining again and again and again. I built this into my Kingdom character of Progesterone, the Queen, who is not satisfied with just reusing the same "room" as she waits for different special guests to arrive each cycle. No! She is very particular and wants to prepare a room that is completely unique for each potential guest. She understands that each guest is different, and there is no way she would allow January's guest to sleep in the room she had prepared for November's guest. This Queen spares no expense and sees no value in thrift. Beyond being merely generous in this level of personal care, our bodies display a superabundant generosity in the level of attention given to the smallest thing.

> *Our bodies are ridiculously generous in providing new endometrial lining again and again and again.*

In this, we can hear an echo of Jesus' words: "Are not five sparrows sold for two pennies? And not one of them is forgotten before God. Why, even the hairs of your head are all numbered. Fear not; you are of more value than many sparrows" (Lk 12:6–7). The intimacy with which God knows and cares for us as individuals is woven throughout all of Scripture. Psalm 139 illustrates this beautifully:

> O Lord, you have searched me and known me!
> You know when I sit down and when I rise up;
>   you discern my thoughts from afar.
> You search out my path and my lying down,
>   and are acquainted with all my ways.
> Even before a word is on my tongue,
>   behold, O Lord, you know it altogether.
> You beset me behind and before,
>   and lay your hand upon me.
> Such knowledge is too wonderful for me;
>   it is high, I cannot attain it. (vv. 1–6)

This is the sort of superabundant attention that is imaged in a very physical way through a woman's menstrual cycle. Women's bodies prepare a completely unique and unrepeatable home for each egg that is released. The sheer amount of work, energy, and skilled coordination of hormones that goes into building up our endometrial lining each cycle should help us reflect on the fact that each and every human person is uniquely created, loved, and cared for by God.

And while the psalmist proceeds to reflect on the way he was knit together in his mother's womb, it is important for us to remember that the radical generosity of a woman's body in providing for human life is performed whether or not she ever conceives and bears a child. Truly, the generosity and the offering of one's body during pregnancy is another reflection of God's parental care for the human person; yet, the biological expense of a menstrual cycle occurs completely independently of a woman's pregnancy intentions, and in many cases still occurs even when there are other difficulties with fertility. It speaks the language of total self-gift for even the mere potential of human life … again and again and again. This character of the feminine genius, reflected in the process of a menstrual cycle, can therefore be appreciated by all women, regardless of our vocational or fertility status. It is a way that our bodies themselves are made to reflect our Creator, simply through our feminine biology.

SUPERABUNDANCE IN QUANTITY AND VOLUME

Oftentimes when we speak of superabundance in God, we think primarily of Jesus' declaration in the Gospel of John: "I came that they may have life, and have it abundantly" (10:10). What does abundance mean, in this case?

Abundance could refer to quantity — to the sheer volume and variety of things that God has made — and to the flourishing of life that he has promised. In particular, we can point to the promise God made to Isaac, to give him "descendants as the stars of heaven" (Gn 26:4). God could have created a single angel, and a single human. He could have made simply one kind of grass, or even a single blade of grass. G. K. Chesterton delights in this abundant creativity of God, likening it to the vitality of a child. Rather than taking for granted the repetition of daisies, for example, as a mere scientific necessity, he states: "It may be that God makes every daisy separately, but has never got tired of making them. It may be that He has the eternal appetite of infancy; for we have sinned and grown old, and our Father is younger than we. The repetition of nature may not be a mere recurrence; it may be a theatrical *encore*."[1]

The superabundant creativity of God fills the earth with a baffling volume and variety of creatures. This is one aspect of having life in abundance, but we see in Scripture that our God is sometimes abundant to the point where it may even begin to appear as waste. Think about the miracle of Jesus feeding the multitude, where God takes what little we have to offer and multiplies it to meet not only our needs, but the needs of our brothers and sisters. This miracle would have been impressive enough if Jesus took the five loaves and two fish, multiplied them, and fed everyone to their fill. But note that Jesus did not just multiply the food to an abundance that was sufficient for our needs: He multiplied to a *superabundance,* such that the leftovers filled a symbolic twelve baskets. This particular miracle was understood to be so important by the early disciples, so representative of Jesus' mission, that it is the only ministerial miracle included in all four Gospels.

From this, we are able to ponder the superabundant way that God generously gives of himself. He is not content to simply fill up what we lack — he desires to give of himself so that we are overflowing. As Paul writes:

But the free gift is not like the trespass. For if many died through the one man's trespass, *much more* have the grace of God and the free gift in the grace of the one man, Jesus Christ, abounded for many. And the free gift is not like the effect of the one man's sin … If, because of the one man's trespass, death reigned through that one man, *much more* will those who receive the abundance of grace and the free gift of righteousness reign in life through the one man Jesus Christ. (Romans 5:15–17, emphasis added)

In other words, abundance of life is also about receiving a super-abundance of God's grace. Gerard Manley Hopkins poetically translated St. Thomas Aquinas's great hymn, *Adoro Te Devote*, to say, "Bathe me, Jesus Lord, in what thy bosom ran / Blood that but one drop of has the pow'r to win / All the world forgiveness of its world of sin."[2] In this hymn, we proclaim that a single drop of Christ's blood would certainly have been sufficient to make up for the trespasses of Adam. St. Julian of Norwich goes even further to offer a meditation on the superabundance of blood that Christ poured forth out of love for us:

The dearworthy blood of our Lord Jesus Christ as verily as it is most precious, so verily it is most plenteous. Behold and see! The precious plenty of his dearworthy blood descended down into hell and burst her bands and delivered all that were there which belonged to the court of heaven. The precious plenty of his dearworthy blood overfloweth all earth, and is ready to wash all creatures of sin. … And evermore it floweth in all heavens enjoying the salvation of all mankind.[3]

We will speak in the next chapter about the connection between period bleeds and Christ's blood; but for now, this image can allow us to reflect on how women who experience very heavy period bleeds may feel a connection to this sort of superabundant outpouring of self.

This also aptly applies to the male reproductive system, in which superabundant quantities (millions upon millions) of sperm are produced, sent forth, and then compete for the sole privilege of fertilizing a single egg. In the system of the man, God's superabundance shows forth in that no expense is spared in quantity or volume. That our bodies would produce such a superabundance of material to facilitate this one action seems to be a microcosm for the superabundant existence God has provided each of us on this earth. Sperm cells are as numerous as the stars in the sky; yet if we were to focus solely on this representation of superabundance, our picture of God would be correct, but severely deficient. When we also focus on the menstrual cycle and the intense care given to a single cell, we also realize the superabundant care God gives to each of us. A woman's egg cells are precious and few. They are like the pearl of great price in Matthew's Gospel (see 13:45–46), a thing so small and yet worth so much to the merchant that he would sell all he had in order to obtain but one.

> In other words, abundance of life is also about receiving a superabundance of God's grace.

The male and female reproductive systems could both image God on their own, but when viewed together, they actually paint a more robust picture of God's superabundance. Specifically, they help us to understand a very peculiar paradox.

I have heard it said that within the family unit, the father is the parent who images God's transcendence — how God is "other" and stands apart from us, even as our loving Father. In a similar way, the mother is the parent who images God's immanence

— how God is "with us" and seems to be a part of us. This sort of complementarity is also what we find in our reproductive systems when we consider abundance: The father represents how God's grace teems forth in creation, while the mother represents how God prepares a place for us, down to the very last detail.

At first, these two aspects of superabundance may seem mutually exclusive of each other. On the one hand, the feminine reflection of superabundant generosity seems to rest in the way a woman's body is designed to pay the utmost attention, and offer the highest and more personal level of care, to a single individual. But we cannot ignore that another aspect of superabundance is found in the idea of multitude, which is reflected better in the masculine reproductive system. These two things appear to compete with each other, because we know from personal experience that we humans are incapable of maintaining intensely intimate relationships with more than just a few people. Yet we insist that God is the Creator of the entire plethora of everything that exists, and also knows each of his individual creations better than they know themselves.

We can close our reflection on superabundance simply by meditating on the beauty of this paradox, as it is expressed through the dual embodiment of God's superabundant generosity in the biology of both woman and man. As the twentieth-century English mystic Caryll Houselander wrote: "[God] does not only give our needs; He is extravagant, almost profligate, in love. Yes … look at the millions of stars, look at the leaves, at the grass, at the daisies, and look at all the countless millions of seeds, wasted, that one take root to be a tree for us! You see … all creation is only one thing, a father clothing and feeding, delighting his child, and saying again and again in everything, 'I am your Father, I love you!'"[4]

CHAPTER 7

The *Imago Dei* in Good Blood

In a previous chapter, we thought about creation, and specifically the human person, as a beautiful work of art that can help us come to know God, the Creator-Artist, more deeply. When it comes to women's cycles, we must admit that there is a part of us that wants to turn away from including our cycles as part of the goodness and beauty of our bodies. I know that for a lot of girls and women, the simple fact that we need to deal with blood on a regular basis is enough to make us uncomfortable, if not completely grossed out. We think to ourselves, "Yes, I am God's image. All my good and beautiful parts are definitely the work of God. But all those other parts that I struggle with — all the ugly parts, or the icky parts, or the inconvenient parts — those are not part of the goodness. All of those things are the result of the Fall." When we think like this, it's easy to imagine that heaven might be a place full of gorgeous models, "perfect" specimens of manhood and womanhood who show us what our "true form" was supposed to take all along.

But are we really sure what parts of us are beautiful and good, and what parts are ugly and icky? To a very large extent, our body image is shaped by the culture around us, whether that's media, shifting cultural norms, or the subjective opinions of the people we love. How do we tease out what is truly, essentially "good" and what we are only taught to think is good? Jesus himself "had no form or comeliness that we should look at him, / and no beauty that we should desire him" (Is 53:2). And yet, we know that Christ — as God — was the personification of truth, goodness, and beauty. How can we reconcile these ideas? If we want to contemplate the goodness of our bodies as a means to coming to know God, then it seems we must divest ourselves of the idea that true goodness and beauty is the same as what society shapes us to think of as good and beautiful.

In particular, this touches very closely to the heart of women's bodies in our reproductive function. A lot of my clients express exasperation and frustration with God that their cycles and periods aren't more straightforward, or that they seem to be experiencing an inordinate amount of suffering related to their menstrual cycles. I do not want to sugarcoat the harsh reality that for many women, our cycles are a place where we can feel particularly broken and abandoned — not just by a medical system, but by the One who designed this system in the first place. However, when we think in this way, we are thinking in the way that humans do, not necessarily as God does. How can we learn to see beauty through his eyes? Can the pain, blood, and mess of our periods be seen in any way as being good?

GOOD BLOOD

To return to the art analogy from previous chapters, I'd like to put forward two scenes that both feature heavily in Christian art: the crucifixion and the Resurrection. It is perhaps easy for us to think about the glory, splendor, beauty, and radiance of the Resurrection. But a fresco of the Resurrection is no better — no more beautiful in its subject matter — than the Pietà.

Indeed, it is precisely through art that the areas of most profound suffering can be transfigured and contemplated in their own unique beauty. A crucifixion scene is not beautiful by earthly standards. It is gross, messy, gory, and heart-wrenchingly painful to look upon. And yet, it is beautiful because it communicates truth: the truth that God chose bodily suffering as his mode of salvation. He spilled his divine blood in order to give us life. If we did not know this truth, our devotion to the crucifix would be macabre, at best. But we know, deep down, that the blood of Christ is different, because it was through this blood that God chose to enact his covenant of salvation with all humankind. This is why, despite the fact that from every human vantage point the day of Jesus' crucifixion was a complete failure, the Bride of Christ insists on calling it good.[1]

How can we learn to see beauty through his eyes? Can the pain, blood, and mess of our periods be seen in any way as being good?

When I teach girls about menarche and what it's like to have a period, the very first thing I tell them is that we need to think about period blood in a completely different way from how we tend to think about other types of blood. Usually, when we see blood, it's a sign that something has gone wrong: We have perhaps fallen and cut ourselves, or are injured in some other way. But period blood is actually a visible sign that a lot of hidden, or relatively invisible, processes have gone exactly right! When we learn all about the complicated symphony of hormones that our body needs to coordinate in order to make up a cycle, we can understand that the period is a sign that our body has been doing a lot of work over the past few weeks and is ready to start over with a new cycle.

I recently had a mom come up to me after a program and thank me for making that point. Her daughter is one of those kids who is really uncomfortable with blood. The sight of it, or even talking about it, can make her feel a little woozy. So her mother (who is a doctor) was a little concerned about how the workshop would go. To this mom's delight and surprise, the re-framing of period blood as "good, healthy blood" helped her daughter feel much more comfortable about the thought of getting a period. They were both optimistic about how this one difference might be able to decrease her worry about menarche when the time came.

I've used this same language to help coach young moms, when the inevitable question pops up of how to explain a period to a curious toddler who insists on accompanying Mom into the bathroom. When your little son or daughter first sees period blood, the natural reaction is for them to worry about Mama's health. So I've found that the most important thing to tell your little kids about periods is that they "are a good, healthy sign that Mama's body is doing just what it needs to do!"

CLEAN AND UNCLEAN

For Catholics, it is not enough to simply assert that period blood is good and healthy from a medical perspective. We need the science to inform our thoughts on the question, but we also have to contend with the fact that Scripture and Tradition have left us a complicated set of stories and ideas pertaining to menstrual blood, with which we need to grapple if there is an aspect of *imago Dei* to be found here. We cannot simply overlook passages because they make us uncomfortable; so before going further, let's tackle some of the most difficult passages front and center: the purity laws of Leviticus. "When a woman has a discharge of blood which is her regular discharge from her body, she shall be in her impurity for seven days. If a woman has a discharge of blood for many days, not at the time of her impurity, or if she has a discharge beyond the time of her impurity, all the days of the discharge she shall continue in uncleanness" (Lv 15:19, 25).

It is important to remember that these lines are preceded by an equal amount of detail explaining the impurity of male emissions, outlining the fact that genital discharge and seminal emission require parallel prohibitions and subsequent purity rites. This also includes the act of sexual intercourse between spouses, which renders both partners "unclean" until the evening and they have bathed.

Here I'd like to pause and give a little bit of clarification on what "clean" and "unclean" indicate with reference to the purity laws of Israel. These designations could be given to objects, animals, or persons, and indicated whether said object, animal, or person was "fit" to participate in proper worship of God. So a jar that was unclean could not be used in a ceremony. An unclean animal (like a pig) could not be sacrificed on the altar. And an unclean person was not adequately prepared to approach God to offer sacrifices or to participate in worship. Some things, like pigs, were inherently unclean and could never be used for worship. Other things, like people, could be rendered temporarily unclean, in which case the person would need to undergo the prescribed purification process in order to be readmitted to communal worship. Rather than cutting them off from God, purity laws were something uniquely gifted to the Jewish people that enabled them to approach God and one another in a way that no other nation was permitted to do. It was through these laws of purity that Israel was given the path to draw closer to the Lord.

So men and women could both experience temporary uncleanliness related to the emission of certain bodily fluids. But this does raise some questions about whether the Bible is putting forward the exact opposite value judgment I am offering. Does the Bible confirm that menstrual blood is bad, by saying that it is "unclean"?

To answer this question, I think it is wise to turn to our modern Jewish sisters who still undertake the rigorous practice of *mikvah* — or ritual cleansing — after their periods. Of course, Jewish women's opinions and comments on this matter will vary just as much as Catholic women's opinions on any number of faith-related topics, but I'd like to share two key insights I received through a survey of modern Jewish literature on the topic:

1. Menstrual purity laws need to be understood in the context of collective Family Purity Law, which explains that the sexual relationship between husband and wife is a spiritual connection in relationship to each other, to children-yet-to-be-conceived, and to God.
2. The words "clean" and "unclean" carry connotations that many modern Jewish women reject, because they are associated with physical dirtiness. Because of this, most women will instead speak of their current status as being "pure" or "impure" before God, in order to reflect the idea that the physical rituals are actually about spiritual realities.

In the book *Mikvah Stories,* Chaya Raichik provides some beautiful commentary that suggests that Jewish women need not see the ritual impurity associated with uterine bleeding as an oppressive or demeaning practice.

> Sometimes there are misconceptions about [the laws of purity], with purity being erroneously translated as "clean" and impure being translated as the opposite of clean. Nothing could be further from the truth. Going to

mikvah is not about becoming "clean," it's about becoming pure and holy. The concept of purity is completely spiritual; it's a dichotomy that *Hashem* invented and only He understands. … Similar to the gaps in a ladder, the time of impurity allows one to pause and refresh before continuing up the next rung and deepening the connection with *Hashem.*[2]

In the context of family purity, a woman's time of *niddah,* or impurity related to uterine bleeding, is seen as a sacred time in which spouses are prohibited from connecting physically with each other so the wife can be intentional about connecting her body and spirit in preparation for deepening her connection with God in the *mikvah* bath, and subsequently with her husband when they resume intercourse. This is echoed and expanded upon by Jewish educator Bonni Goldberg, who writes:

I was also completely perplexed about how the *Niddah* laws could be interpreted by feminists as a sexist and degrading patriarchal move. … Historically, in a time and place when women were commonly considered the property of men who could require sex from their wives at will … timing of the monthly hiatus was dictated by the woman's cycle, in effect by the woman herself, not only while she was bleeding, but for a whole seven days afterwards. And only she could signal the end of the separation period, because only she knew how long she bled. … Doesn't that sound like a practice devised by women rather than men?[3]

Of course, we believe that Jewish ritual purity laws were devised neither by men or women, but by God himself — and in the earliest days of the Church, the Council of Jerusalem confirmed that

Christians need not follow Mosaic purity laws since Jesus fulfilled the law and opened up the grace of salvation to all through himself (see Acts 15:1–35). But it is nonetheless important for us, as modern Catholic women, to listen to the perspectives of our Jewish sisters who are able to speak to us directly from the experience of *mikvah,* to help us wrestle with any negative things we have assumed about our own bodies through the Scriptures.

Particularly, meditating on the *mikvah* and the concept of cleanliness through ritual washing should help us wrestle with the very real fact that periods are … messy. Quite literally, our periods do stain things. Blood gets everywhere sometimes. And especially for women with heavy periods, or for girls and women who lack the basic menstrual care supplies needed to keep their blood from getting everywhere, it's easy to see how our minds might confuse the physical desire for cleanliness with our spiritual state and our relationship to God. The *mikvah* is an intentional time when Jewish women prepare both the physical and spiritual cleansing of their bodies for the dual purpose of worship and for relationship with their spouse. Now that we are no longer bound by purity laws, Christians have the opportunity to see how blood does not separate our bodies from God — it profoundly unites us. But the process of *mikvah* can help us realize that even from the beginning, God has never excluded our bodies from his desire for relationship with us.[4]

> *Now that we are no longer bound by purity laws, Christians have the opportunity to see how blood does not separate our bodies from God — it profoundly unites us*

Having thus shown how the biological concept of the "good period blood" can harmonize with our understanding of God's stance toward menstruation, we can thus proceed to discuss the ways in which our menstrual bleeding can be understood to *image* God. In previous chapters, I have tried to keep the entire cycle as the primary focus, but here we are really focusing on a single element of a woman's cycle: her period. This is the time when our cycle symptoms are most external and visible — and, as we have stated, is really the only thing we knew for certain about cycles until relatively recently in medicine.

BLOOD: PARADOX OF LIFE AND DEATH

In the Bible, blood appears often as a particular form of sacrifice. "For the life of the flesh is in the blood; and I have given it for you upon the altar to make atonement for your souls; for it is the blood that makes atonement, by reason of the life" (Lv 17:11). These instructions are given in the context of God explaining how the Israelites are to eat their food — that is, they are permitted to eat the flesh of animals, but they may not eat the blood. The reason given is that blood is equal to life, and therefore is reserved for a very special purpose: atonement.

The offering of an animal's blood on the altar is meant to symbolically represent the offering of the sinner's blood — a pouring out of his or her life as an act of reparation to God who is the giver of life. In this type of sacrifice, the blood of the animal substitutes for the blood of the person. The blood of the animal poured out is a symbol of death, a signifier of a person who is willing to "die" to their sins.

Yet we read in Exodus of a different sort of animal sacrifice that has nothing to do with atonement. In preparation for the final plague, God tells Moses to instruct the Israelites to procure an unblemished lamb and sacrifice it:

> They shall take some of the blood, and put it on the two
> doorposts and the lintel of the houses in which they eat
> them. In this manner you shall eat it: your loins girded,

> your sandals on your feet, and your staff in your hand;
> and you shall eat it in haste. It is the Lord's Passover. For
> I will pass through the land of Egypt that night, and I
> will strike all the first-born in the land of Egypt, both
> man and beast, and on all the gods of Egypt I will exe-
> cute judgments: I am the Lord. The blood shall be a sign
> for you, upon the houses where you are; and when I see
> the blood, I will pass over you, and no plague shall fall
> upon you to destroy you, when I strike the land of Egypt.
> (12:7, 11–13)

In this text, there is no mention that the blood of the paschal
lamb will atone for anyone's sins. The slaughter of the animal
is not indicated to be an act of reparation; it is instead an act
of salvation through ransom. As Melito of Sardis stated in the
second century, "[Christ] ransomed us from our servitude to
the world, as he had ransomed Israel from the hand of Egypt;
he freed us from our slavery to the devil, as he had freed Israel
from the hand of Pharaoh."[5] Destruction is coming, and the only
thing that can save a household from certain death is to mark
the dwelling with a sign God has ordained — the sign of blood.

In some way, we could think of the lamb substituting for
the life of the firstborn — the lamb was slain and therefore the
firstborn was spared. However, it is important to note that unlike sacrifices of atonement, guilt is not the reason the firstborn
was slain. The plagues were meant to be signs for Pharaoh, to
demonstrate God's power and the favored status of his people
Israel. "The Egyptians shall know that I am the Lord," God tells
Moses, "when I stretch forth my hand upon Egypt and bring
out the sons of israel from among them" (Ex 7:5). Therefore,
the blood of the lamb was also intended to be a sign — both
to Pharaoh and to the Angel of Death — an efficacious sign by
which the Israelites traded the life of a lamb for the salvation of

their firstborn sons, and ultimately, their entire nation. Salvation through blood is therefore a paradox, because unlike the blood of atonement in which the physical death of the animal is the symbolic death of the person, the blood of salvation is an actual death that represents — and even bestows — life.

Speaking about the Passover, St. John Chrysostom wrote, "If we were to ask [Moses] what he meant, and how the blood of an irrational beast could possibly save men endowed with reason, his answer would be that the saving power lies not in the blood itself, but in the fact that it is a sign of the Lord's blood."[6] Our Church possesses and hands down a rich theology regarding the saving blood of Christ, beyond what we can cover here. The one point we must make is that in the person of Jesus Christ, these dual elements of atonement and salvation — blood signifying both death *and* life — are wedded together in the blood of Good Friday.

This theology is placed front and center at the beginning of John's Gospel, when John the Baptist proclaims, "Behold, the Lamb of God, who takes away the sin of the world!" (1:29). In John's Gospel, Jesus is clearly depicted as the Passover lamb, yet it's possible that a Jewish reader would have been struck by the oddity of the baptist's phrase, because according to Exodus, the Passover lamb did not take away sins. I find it easy to imagine how the baptist could have been seen as a little bit of a nut: People would probably often wonder, *"What is he talking about?"* Of course, we know that John was a prophet. Somehow he knew that Jesus' blood is not only distinct because it is God's blood offered on the cross, but also because it is a perfect sacrifice that both atones and saves.

Strictly speaking, we must insist that there is nothing about women's menstrual blood that either atones for sin or offers salvation from death. And yet we do see how menstrual blood, as a unique form of human blood that is able to be shed in abundance without leading to death, is a sort of *sign* of both the life and death that is uniquely expressed through the sacrificial blood of Christ. The blood of Good Friday and the good blood of periods are not one and the same — but they do rhyme. A woman's menstrual blood holds a unique place in human life, just as Christ's blood holds a unique place in God's divine economy.

One passage in Genesis illustrates this point and perhaps prefigures the idea that menstrual blood can image the blood of Christ: the episode of Rachel and the household idols.

Rachel was the beloved wife of Jacob, who was later named "Israel" and whose sons represented the twelve tribes. Jacob was also married to Rachel's older sister, Leah, but only because he had been tricked into marrying Leah by Laban, the girls' father. In our particular story of interest, Jacob is told by God to flee from his father-in-law, Laban, to go back to the land of his ancestors. The two men had reached a point of contention in their already strained relationship, so Jacob packs up his household and decides to flee. For some unknown reason, Rachel decides to abscond with her father's household idols and keeps this a secret from her husband. When Laban catches up with them and demands that his stolen idols be returned, Jacob rashly responds that Laban can search the whole camp for the idols — if they are discovered, the one who stole them should be put to death.

This is a moment of pure dramatic tension: Jacob is completely unaware that the trajectory of the entire nation of Israel hangs in the balance with these stupid household idols. If Rachel were to be put to death, not only would Jacob lose his beloved wife, but Benjamin, the beloved youngest son, also would never be born. As Joseph's only full brother, Benjamin plays a crucial role in the re-unification of Joseph with the rest of his family at the end of Genesis, which allows them to survive the great famine through the hospitality of the pharaoh and become the nation of Israel. The reader, who presumably knows about the rest of the story, understands that under no circumstances can Jacob make good on this foolish oath!

It is here that menstrual blood plays a somewhat surprising role. Laban begins searching the camp, and we read: "Now Rachel had taken the household gods and put them in the camel's saddle, and sat upon them. Laban felt all about the tent, but did not find them. And she said to her father, 'Let not my lord be angry that I cannot rise before you, for the way of women is upon me.' So he searched, but did not find the household gods" (31:34–35).

Whether Rachel was actually experiencing her period is uncertain, but we do know that she used menstruation as a means to intentionally hoodwink her father and, consequently, save her own life. In this way, menstrual blood — either in fact or merely in symbol — serves as the device through which God's plan of covenant fulfillment is able to remain intact. By the menstrual blood of a woman, the legacy of Israel, which was so foolishly jeopardized by Jacob's indignation, is secured. Here we see a prefiguration of the paradox of blood, made manifest in Christ: The shedding of blood is able to divert what seems like inevitable destruction.

BLOOD AS FOOD

When we think of the blood of Christ, it is paramount that we do not overlook the Real Presence of Christ's body, blood, soul and divinity in the Eucharist. Is there any connection between menstruation and the Eucharistic species of Christ's blood? The resounding answer given by the Church is yes — and we see this in one very specific image of the Blessed Virgin Mary that dates back to at least the sixth century and remained popular in both medieval and Renaissance piety: the *Virgo Lactans,* or Nursing Madonna.

In this image of mother and child, the infant Christ is seen either reaching for or suckling at the breast of his mother. It is a very intimate and human image, which allows us to reflect on the personal connection shared between Mary and her Son; but it is also an image rich in theological significance for our conversation here, because according to medieval medicine, milk was actually produced through the transfiguration of menstrual blood. Without a proper understanding of the menstrual cycle and its hormones, medievals believed that the body of a child was formed in utero directly out of a woman's blood, just as Adam was formed from the dust of the earth. So blood in the woman's body was first built up into the form of the child. After birth, blood was transformed into milk to provide nourishment for the child — to give the child life.[7] This is the medieval explanation for why women don't experience periods while they are nursing! One seventh-century explanation reads:

> Lac (milk) derives its name from its color, because it is a white liquor, for the Greeks call white λευκός and its nature is changed from blood; for after the birth whatever blood has not yet been spent in nourishing the womb flows by a natural passage to the breasts, and whitening by their virtue, receives the quality of milk.[8]

To drive home the imagery, though, we can look at the source of milk: the breast — or in other words, the woman's side. This idea that milk was blood, transformed into food, flowing from the side, was in turn seen as a symbol for the Eucharist — the source and summit of the life of the Church, of which Mary was the perfect archetype.

Thus, a lactating Mary was an image that carried immensely rich symbolism. It represented the humanity of Christ by showing his reliance upon Mary's flesh and blood for his own sustenance. The nursing Madonna drew viewers into contemplation of the blood of Christ, given through our Mother Church, as true sustenance for our own souls. The image also puts Mary, as the biological mother and nurturer of Christ, in the role of supreme intercessor because it shows how her Son chooses to cling to her maternal care.

CATHOLIC WOMEN AND THE STIGMATA

One final idea I would like to put forward for reflection is the connection between women and another sort of bleeding — that of the stigmata, or the bleeding wounds of Christ. The word *stigmata* is taken from Paul's Letter to the Galatians, in which he writes, "Henceforth let no man trouble me; for I bear on my body the marks of Jesus" (6:17). It is unknown whether Saint Paul literally meant that he bore the wounds of Christ, but we do know that since the twelfth century, confirmed cases of stigmata have been demonstrated in which the hands, feet, sides, or sometimes the head of a holy person will bleed in imitation of the wounds of Christ. Saint Bonaventure records this phenomenon occurring in the life of Saint Francis, after he beheld a seraphic vision:

> As the vision disappeared, it left in his heart a marvelous ardor and imprinted on his body markings that were no less marvelous. Immediately the marks of the nails began to appear in his hands and feet just as he had seen a little before in the figure of the man crucified. His hands and feet seemed to be pierced through the center by nails … also his right side, as if pierced with a lance, was marked with a red wound from which his sacred blood often flowed.[9]

A more modern saint who experienced the same wounds was St. Pio of Pietrelcina, also known as Padre Pio. Yet, when we survey the history of stigmata in the Church, we see that at least eighty percent of reported stigmatists are women. By some estimates, the number skews to higher than ninety percent.[10] Women such as St. Catherine of Siena, St. Gemma Galgani, St. Rita of Cascia, St. Catherine de Ricci, and St. Frances of Rome are merely a few of the female saints who have experienced stigmata, either visibly or invisibly (as in the case of St. Catherine of Siena, whose wounds only became known after her death). In addition to being experienced primarily by women, the wounds of stigmata also tend to have periodic cycles, meaning that blood is not flowing from the wounds all the time. In some cases, the wounds may disappear for weeks at a time, only to reappear again later.[11] Is there some meaning to be gleaned from the fact that this holy bleeding is experienced so predominantly by women?

Historian Caroline Walker Bynum suggests that especially for medieval women, the supernatural excretion of stigmatic blood was seen as a sort of fulfillment of the natural excretion of menstrual blood. She observes that "holy women were often said neither to eat nor excrete. Stigmatists or myroblytes were often miraculous fasters ... and theologians underlined the fact that those who bled or exuded unusual fluids did not excrete in the ordinary ways."[12] We know, and the medievals understood as well, that depleting key nutrients from our bodies through fasting can produce a state of amenorrhea in women, so there is certainly a natural cause that can be discerned here between holy fasts and lack of periods. However, in the case of many holy women, there is also plenty of evidence that supernatural causes are at work. According to Pope St. John Paul II's account, "medical doctors remained baffled"[13] by the curious case of Blessed Alexandrina Maria da Costa, who subsisted on nothing but the Eucharist for more than thirteen years. So while we must tread carefully in the Church so as not to glamorize disordered relationships with food, we also can admit that God sometimes calls individuals to witness to his complete providence in radical, confounding ways — particularly when it comes to this apparent supernatural relationship between women and bleeding.

The stigmata is certainly a unique and sometimes challenging spiritual gift for us to understand. A number of questions and controversies surrounding stigmata have surfaced over the centuries, but our Church does recognize it in some few cases, so it is worthy of consideration when reflecting on how women's periods may image God. The connection between the natural bleeding of menses, and the supernatural bleeding experienced through the miraculous appearance of the wounds of Christ, tells us that in Catholic theology, the mere act of bleeding itself is in no way profane. In fact, we can see that through association with and imitation of Christ, prolonged and cyclical bleeding can become a participation in the very life of God. It might even be considered a predominantly, if supernaturally speaking not exclusively, feminine participation.

Thus, rather than seeing our natural menstrual blood as a part of the "curse" of Eve, as Catholic women we are invited to reconsider our periods as a physical, natural, and embodied reflection — or *image* — of the good, salvific blood of Christ.

CHAPTER 8

Cycles, Mary, and the *Imago Dei*

In theology, it's very easy to look at a person — for example, Jesus Christ — and to speak in a very deep way about the theological significance of certain points of doctrine pertaining to that person. For example, Jesus Christ is both God and man. Theologians — in fact, entire ecumenical councils — have debated how Christ's humanity and divinity exist together in a single person. As a Church, we have debated how many wills Jesus has and the implications of that conversation. Yet as important as these theological debates are, we still have to remember that we're speaking about a person — and a person is never merely the sum of a series of statements. I cannot sum up my children by simply telling you their favorite color, their favorite cereal, and what they like to do each day; a person is much more complicated than that.

Likewise, because of the privileged place Mary holds in theology, it can be very easy for us to create a series of abstract statements about who we understand Mary to be and be comfortable leaving it at that. We should articulate the fact that Mary is the Mother of God. Catholics should understand her role in salvation history as the second Eve, in parallel with the fact that Christ is the second Adam.[1] We need to understand that "the knot of Eve's disobedience was loosed by the obedience of Mary."[2] We need to profess and contemplate the dogmatic pronouncements from the Church that confirm that Mary was conceived without sin and was assumed body and soul into heaven. Going beyond that, we can also assert certain things about how she functions as an archetype, meaning that she is the symbolic embodiment of the Church (see *Lumen Gentium*, 53, 63) and of "woman."

But among all of these important things that we need to say about Mary, we also cannot lose sight of the fact that she is a biological, human woman. She exists and lives and reigns in heaven at this moment in her female body. Being the Mother of God wasn't an abstract theological concept for Miryam of Nazareth. It meant getting up each morning and tending to the necessary duties of feeding, clothing, and even bathing a boy child named Jesus. It meant looking upon the eyes of her child and remembering the dance of this same child in her womb. It also meant knowing that her own flesh and blood were torn apart at his death. Our theological statements must never eclipse the fact that Mary experienced life as a female human, body and soul.

As we conclude our theological reflections on women's cycles, it's fitting to bring everything to a culmination with Mary, since she is conceptually and actually femininity, par excellence. Yet in doing so, we are faced with some questions about what that could mean with respect to the biological functions of her female body. Much earlier in this text, I alluded to work that suggests that being conceived without sin would mean that Mary's reproductive system worked differently from what we understand about female biological function. With deference to our beloved Mother Church — understanding that this is an open question for theological speculation and my readers are free to disregard my opinions — I'd like to make the case that it is not only fitting, but also theologically significant, for us to entertain the idea that Mary might have had menstrual cycles and periods just like every other woman. After that, we will contemplate some very specific ties Mary has to images of cycles in our Faith, which add depth and complexity to our concept of how our female bodies *image* God.

THE FITTINGNESS OF MARY'S MENSTRUATION

On the surface, it appears that certain theological statements about Mary create points of tension when we think about her biological womanhood. In particular, the dogma of the Immaculate Conception states:

> We declare, pronounce, and define that the doctrine which holds that the most Blessed Virgin Mary, in the first instance of her conception, by a singular grace and privilege granted by Almighty God, in view of the merits of Jesus Christ, the Savior of the human race, was preserved free from all stain of original sin, is a doctrine revealed by God and therefore to be believed firmly and constantly by all the faithful. (*Ineffabilis Deus*, Pope Pius IX)

What does Mary's sinlessness mean for her experience of embodied life on this planet? This is a bit of a different question from simply asking, "What was it like for Adam and Even in the Garden of Eden?" While Adam and Eve experienced their sinless state in a likewise prelapsarian world, Mary's experience of sinlessness was lived in a world already fallen. What could that possibly have been like? From what we know in the Bible, we can say that being conceived without sin did not insulate Mary from the political troubles of the day. She was still subjected to the Roman authorities. She was subject to grief and sorrow as her Son willingly entered into suffering on our behalf. Can any of this tell us about what she experienced in her sinless body? Which bodily events are simply inherent to finite matter, and which ones are weaknesses brought about by the Fall?

One of the weirder, but potentially more interesting questions I asked as a child was whether Jesus and Mary ever needed to go to the bathroom. The logic went like this: If they didn't experience original sin, that means their bodies and souls were perfect and worked perfectly together. Therefore, it's at least theoretically possible that their digestive systems worked perfectly without any "waste." Yet even as a child, I came to the conclusion that it would be absolutely absurd to insist that the Son of God, as a male human, never had to pee.

I could conceive of a transfigured, resurrected body, which was capable of walking through walls and doors, and appearing differently in such a way that even Mary Magdalene wouldn't have recognized him immediately after the Resurrection (see Jn 20:11–18). I could imagine that Resurrected Jesus would be able to eat fish with his apostles on the shore without his glorified body needing to perform all of the mundane bodily functions associated with digestion. And I came to this conclusion because I understood resurrection to be something that changed the human body into something qualitatively and experientially different than it had ever been before. Some of these activities have traditionally been attributed to the fact the Jesus' resurrected body is uniquely connected to the Godhead (like, walking through walls). But some other activities (like, eating without the biological need for nutrition) seem to be a part of glorified human nature itself.

To put it a little differently, a glorified body is not just a better body; it's a different mode, so to speak, of the human body. Glorified bodies are not made for life on earth — they are made for eternal life in heaven. Thomas Aquinas explains that one main difference between earthly and heavenly existence is that heaven will have no purpose for basic acts of generation and nutrition. God's command to "Be fruitful and multiply" in Genesis will have already been fulfilled. "In the state of the resurrection," explains Aquinas, "the human race will already have the number of individuals preordained by God."[3] So there is clearly a distinction to be made even between Adam and Eve's embodied existence in Eden and embodied existence in the New Jerusalem. The *Catechism* echoes this distinction between earthly and heavenly life: "Christ is raised with his own body: 'See my hands and my feet, that it is I myself'; but he did not return to an earthly life. So, in him, 'all of them will rise again with their own bodies which they now bear,' but Christ 'will change our lowly body to be like his glorious body,' into a 'spiritual body'" (999).

Thus, even if I could conceive of a glorified human body that never produced excrement, here on Earth — in this life — it just doesn't seem fitting. It's important to remember that the restoration of humanity and the culmination of God's plan for salvation is different from the beginning of humanity. Heaven is not simply going back to the Garden of Eden. Heaven is the New Jerusalem, which is something qualitatively and experientially different — a new mode, so to speak, of existing with God. Hildegard von Bingen explains this when she says, "Thus Man, having been delivered, shines in God, and God in Man; Man, having community with God, has in Heaven more radiant brightness than he had before. This would not have been so if the Son of God had not put on flesh, for if Man had remained in Paradise, the Son of God would not have suffered on the cross."[4]

This is echoed again in the Office of Readings for Holy Saturday, where we read from the ancient homily: "Rise, let us leave this place. The enemy led you out of the earthly paradise. I will not restore you to that paradise, but I will enthrone you in heaven."[5]

As we meditate on Mary, we can hold on to the fact that even though she was conceived without sin, we don't need to say that her body functioned on this planet as if she were already in heavenly glory. We know, for a fact, that in heaven there will be no suffering. But clearly, Mary and Jesus were both capable of suffering in this life, despite their sinless nature. We know that they ate and slept and wept here on Earth.

So it makes sense for us to suggest that Mary's digestive system worked as we expect a typical digestive system to work. And we can therefore give ourselves permission to consider that Mary's body might have functioned just as we would expect a biologically female woman's body to function in her menstrual cycle as well. In other words, it is not unfitting to suggest that the same body that ovulated, gestated, and lactated to give life to Our Lord could also have ovulated and menstruated the rest of the time.

Why is this important? First, because whatever is said of Mary is said because of what it reveals to us about Christ. We insist that she was actually, truly pregnant with Jesus and contributed her own egg to be divinely fertilized, because we need to profess that Jesus was actually incarnate as a *human*. St. Gregory of Nazianzus says this very clearly:

> If anyone does not believe that Holy Mary is the Mother of God, he is severed from the Godhead. If anyone should assert that He passed through the Virgin as through a channel, and was not at once divinely and humanly formed in her (divinely, because without the

intervention of a man; humanly, because in accordance with the laws of gestation), he is in like manner godless.[6]

Therefore, if we allow our theological formulations to drift our concept of Jesus and Mary's body-soul existence too far from our own human experience, we run the risk of downplaying the importance of Jesus entering into human life not just *for* us but *with* us in every way except for sin.

In the Letter to the Hebrews we read, "We have not a high priest who is unable to sympathize with our weaknesses, but one who in every respect has been tempted as we are, yet without sinning" (Heb 4:15), which is echoed in the Mass, in the text of Eucharistic Prayer IV: "And you so loved the world, Father most holy, that in the fullness of time you sent your Only Begotten Son to be our Savior. Made incarnate by the Holy Spirit and born of the Virgin Mary, he shared our human nature in all things but sin."[7]

In other words, it is not unfitting to suggest that the same body that ovulated, gestated, and lactated to give life to Our Lord could also have ovulated and menstruated the rest of the time.

Christ, in his sinless body, assumed even the possibility of death. If this is important to assert about our Savior, it should mean that any attempt we make to isolate Mary from the normal functions of bodily life should be done with great hesitation, especially based on what we know about the incredible importance of menstrual cycle hormones to women's health. Could God have preserved Mary's bodily health without her cycles? Of course. But it would also be very fitting of God to allow his mother's body to proceed according to the wise design for female health that he designed for women in the beginning.

The other reason I believe it is theologically important for us to not erase Mary's cycles from our contemplation is because of the dimension of sign, which we have been speaking of this entire time. Our bodies are *images* of God, meant to direct us to our own holiness and to the contemplation of God through his likeness in our selves as male and female. The previous chapters have made a case for how our cycles can truly function as *signs* that point us toward a deeper understanding of God through the female body. Is it possible that God withheld this particular dimension of *sign* from Mary's body because it was already fulfilled in some other way? Of course. But if he did do this, it is an aspect of his intimate relationship with Mary that remains hidden from us in this life.

THE HIDDEN IMAGE

I would like to pivot in our reflections toward this concept of "hiddenness," which is itself an element of God's image. "*Adoro te devote, latens Deitas,*"[8] sings the heart of St. Thomas Aquinas. The invisible God hides himself in the elements of bread and wine in the Eucharist. We look upon him with our eyes, yet his mysterious presence is veiled.

In so many ways, God hides in plain sight. And we see this lived out in the mystifyingly quiet, hidden life of the Holy Family, especially Mary. St. Louis de Montfort writes:

> Mary was singularly hidden during her life. It is on this account that the Holy Ghost and the Church call her *Alma Mater* — "Mother secret and hidden." Her humility was so profound that she had no inclination on earth more powerful or more constant than that of hiding herself, from herself as well as from every other creature, so as to be known to God only.[9]

There is a great contrast between Mary's hiddenness, which is sought out in order to preserve intimacy with God, and the hiddenness that Adam and Eve choose because they were ashamed of their nakedness before God. In the latter, we have what amounts to an escape attempt — trying to hide from God in order to get away from him. God is "over there" and so we must hide "over here." But Mary's hiddenness is the sort that could only be possible with the Incarnate God, a hiddenness that does not suggest God is "over there" but is "with us here."

Menstrual cycles are, for the most part, completely absent in the writings of our holy fathers and mothers. With a few exceptions, it is a topic that is almost completely hidden — which begs the question of whether menstrual cycles have been hidden like Mary, in order to be known and experienced as a radical intimacy with God, or whether they are hidden like Adam and Eve, who were ashamed and afraid of that intimacy in their current state.

I'm inclined to believe that this is a both/and sort of situation. Perhaps it is the case that for most of our forebears, the topic of menstrual cycle has been an uncomfortable or even shame-inducing thing to speak about. We haven't quite been sure what to say or how to understand them. But I will also venture a guess that many holy women did not write about these things because they did experience something intimate and mystical with God through this bodily function, which was preserved by keeping it to themselves rather than subjecting it to the scrutiny of others who might not understand. St. Teresa of Ávila explains that this secret enjoyment and the impulse to hide from public knowledge of their experience is something many holy people have when they are given a spiritual gift: "When this favor is granted them in secret, their esteem for it is great … For these persons know the malice of the world, and they understand that the world will not perhaps regard their experience for what it is, but that what the Lord should be praised for will perhaps be the occasion for rash judgments."[10]

And now it strikes me as profoundly fitting that the science of our menstrual cycles should remain so relatively hidden until such a time as ours, when culture's very understanding of the nature of man and woman is so broken and confused. Precisely when society is asking, "What *is* a woman?" it is as if Truth is breaking through the confusion to explain that "woman" is an integration of external sex characteristics with a rich, cyclical interior life. What could have remained hidden before must now be brought to light, in order to draw souls to Christ. We can see this echoed also through the person of Mary, who was not permitted to remain hidden, but instead has been elevated to the throne of heaven, as our beloved Queen.

In the last century, Pope John Paul II proclaimed: "'Woman' is the representative and the archetype of the whole human race: she represents the humanity which belongs to all human beings, both men and women" (*Mulieris Dignitatem*, 4). This is, of course, signified par excellence in the person of Mary, but note that John Paul II did not say that Mary, exclusively, is the archetype of the whole human race. He said, "woman." And so, at the conclusion of this section, I'd like to invite you to contemplate certain aspects of Mary as "woman" — even if she did not have menstrual cycles — that are reflected or signaled through our own cycle experience.

Another way of saying this is that I'd like all of us to think about how menstrual cycles are "womanly," even if that means that they are a mere signal in this life of the fulfillment of glorified womanhood yet to come.

CYCLICAL SIGNS POINTING TOWARD MARY

The Moon — The word "menstruation" comes from the Latin term *menses,* which is simply the plural of "month," a word that traditionally marks the measure of one moon to the next. We have stated before that women don't need to have 28-day cycles in order to be considered "regular," but this linguistic thread traces the similarity between a 29.5-day lunar cycle and a typical length for a woman's menstrual cycle.

Last year, I spoke with a woman who had been a cycle educator for many years. She confided to me that when she first got her period as a young teen, she kept a secret little notebook and tried to track her cycles with the moon. Intuitively, she felt that there was a connection between this lesser heavenly body and her own female body. "But," she laughed as she reminisced, "I never saw any connection. It was a nice thought, though!" There is no scientific proof that women's cycles are directly related in any sort of causal relationship to phases of the moon, but that lack of proof does not negate the fact that many ancient cultures just assumed the connection. In short, the identity of "woman" was very much tied into the presence and activity of the moon. Our modern-day knowledge of cycles can go one step further in this imagery, since we can also now speak of phases within the cycle, just as we speak about phases of the moon.

> *Mary's connection with the moon stands as a sign, or perhaps an invitation, for all humanity to emulate: We must all seek to be little moons, reflecting the Light of Christ to the world.*

What is the connection with Mary? Archbishop Fulton Sheen summed up centuries of Christian imagery connecting Mary with the moon when he wrote:

> God, Who made the sun, also made the moon. The moon does not take away from the brilliance of the sun. The moon would be only a burnt-out cinder floating in the immensity of space were it not for the sun. All its light is reflected from the sun. The Blessed Mother reflects her Divine Son; without him, she is nothing. With

him, she is the Mother of Men. On dark nights we are
grateful for the moon; when we see it shining, we know
there must be a sun.[11]

Here we see that Mary's connection with the moon stands as a
sign, or perhaps an invitation, for all humanity to emulate: We
must all seek to be little moons, reflecting the Light of Christ to
the world. This helps us remember that an image is not the same
as a copy. We bear some meaningful resemblance to our Creator,
but any light or goodness we reflect is due to the fact that we
receive it as a gift from our Source. Thus, we can contemplate
the weaving together of all of these signs: menstruation connects
"woman" to the moon, which is perfectly fulfilled in the person
of Mary, and serves as a sign for all of us — male and female —
to imitate as creatures in relationship to our Creator.

The Circle of Beads — The first time I was ever shown a set of
Cycle Beads, I thought it was a strange version of the Rosary —
or perhaps some chaplet — that I had never seen. It was then
explained to me that this circular string of colored beads was
used by women all over the world for family planning with a
method known as the Standard Days Method. This is a variation
of the rhythm method, which was developed by the Institute for
Reproductive Health at Georgetown. At this point, "beads" can
be tracked on an app, but when it was initially developed in the
early 2000s, it was literally a set of beads. Each bead represented
one cycle day: The red bead marked the first day of your period, which was then followed by brown beads, white beads that
indicated potentially fertile days, and then more brown beads
marking the likely infertile days at the end of the cycle. A woman would slide a small rubber ring around the beads in order to
track her cycle and fertility status, going around the circle and
returning to the red bead when her next bleed started.

When I give talks to young Catholic women about body literacy, I often include a side-by-side image of Cycle Beads and a rosary and ask them what this resonance stirs up for them. This is not a theological exercise, meant to elicit any particular doctrinal points about Mary and cycles, but rather an opportunity to invite curiosity and contemplation. Here are a few things women have shared in those moments:[12]

> *"The red bead is kind of like the crucifix on the rosary: it's where you start and where you end up."*

> *"It's like women's bodies are a template for the spirituality that Our Lady wants to share with us."*

> *"A circle is a pretty common shape. I know other religions have similar prayer aids. But when you see them side by side like this, it makes me think that there's a sort of mystery here about women and prayer and our bodies. I need to sit with this idea longer."*

> *"The Cycle Beads track the passing of days in a woman's life. It makes me think about how the Rosary tracks the passing of days and years in one particular woman's life."*

> *"The Rosary is a contemplative prayer. You're not supposed to speed through it, but to really focus on each decade and think about what it means. Maybe the cycle beads show us how we can be intentional about slowing down and really thinking about the meaning of the different cycle phases we go through as women."*

Let us therefore take Mary as our model, so that we can ponder all these things about our female bodies in our heart. As a first-century woman, Miryam of Nazareth didn't know much about menstrual cycles, but we are told that after the very stressful event of going three days without knowing where her Son was in Jerusalem, she was reunited with him and "kept all these things in her heart" (Lk 2:51). She models contemplation for us, which is to simply allow ourselves to think about what God has done and is doing in our lives, and to be open to the presence of God.

Another word for image is the Greek word *eikon*, or icon. We have been speaking of the "image" of God expressed through women's cycles, but now we have an invitation to also consider the body like an icon: an image that actually leads us through contemplation to an encounter of the Divine. St. John Damascene says that holy images (icons) are things that actually "sanctify the sight … imperceptibly [introducing] my soul to the glory of God."[13]

Taking Mary as our example, let us therefore ponder these things in our heart as we behold our own image, letting it traverse from our eyes into our hearts, to the core of our being, to speak to us of the presence of God.

CHAPTER 9

Getting Started with Cycle Charting

For the theological concepts we've discussed so far, it really doesn't make much of a difference whether a woman understands the "hidden" biology of her cycle or not. A woman can learn to reflect on her cycles as part of her *imago Dei* simply by experiencing her bleeds and feeling the cyclical changes in her body, even if she doesn't fully understand what they are telling her. This is right and proper, because for the vast majority of human history, our experience of cycles has been limited to this!

But now we can ask ourselves, as twenty-first century women: what would it add to my understanding of myself if I were to learn how to "read" my cycles in a more detailed and intimate way? The rest of our book will focus on answering this particular question, which is really all about putting the theory of our theological reflection into practice through cycle charting.

Before we begin, though, it's prudent for me to give you permission, as a reader, not to agonize over either the previous theological section or all of the following things we are going to discuss. For many women, simply learning how to reframe our cycles as "good" through a theological lens is going to take a lot of time. You may want to sit with this idea and pray about it before moving into any attempt at practical applications.

> *When you commit to trying to understand a part of Creation through the lens of faith — no matter how small — it is not very long before you begin to encounter a sense of unfathomable mystery about it.*

Conversely, maybe the theological reflection felt overwhelming, and you just really want to get to the practical considerations. After all, the vast majority of women who have learned about their cycles have done so for one very practical reason: to use this information for family planning. Most of my clients have not thought deeply about their cycles as mirrors of the liturgical life of the Church. They simply appreciate the value and the utility of the information for their particular goals, and perhaps begin to ask deeper questions after they have been charting for many years.

I also want to very clear that nothing about this text is intended to be prescriptive. My goal is not to tell you that you *should* experience your cycles in a certain way, or change your life to align with your cycle in any particular way, or attach any specific spirituality to your practice of cycle charting. I am not here to tell you that you *should* apply knowledge about your cycles to all of the areas of life we are about to discuss. To be perfectly blunt, there are also plenty of situations in which I think it prudent for women *not* to chart their cycles. I simply want to open up the space for Catholic women to contemplate this aspect of our unique female biology.

In Teresa of Avila's masterwork *The Interior Castle*, in the midst of her explanation on how the soul journeys towards God through prayer, she simply states, "Even in our own selves there are great secrets that we don't understand." This precisely echoes the sentiment I have felt unfolding throughout the years as I have gone deeper into my work as a cycle educator. When you commit to trying to understand a part of Creation through the lens of faith — no matter how small — it is not very long before you begin to encounter a sense of unfathomable mystery about it. So this is merely an invitation, one among many invitations God extends to us throughout our lives, to consider the marvelous way God has made us, and how understanding His design can help us be more fully ourselves.

We should be careful, in the following chapters, not to conflate the chart and the person. When we chart our cycles, we are simply accumulating data about our biology and then putting that information in conversations with other aspects of our lives. Your menstrual cycle chart may tell you important things about your biology, but it's not some fortune-telling crystal ball. A chart cannot tell us about who we are as people, because it is simply a visual representation of data. The human element — which is also part of our *imago Dei* — is the ability to contextualize the data and bring meaning out of it for our lives, our situations, and our relationships.

In order to dive into these aspects of ourselves which can be explored through cycle charting, it would first be helpful for us to take a step back and look at the process of learning to "read" our cycles. What exactly does it entail? What information will I get? What options are available if I want to learn?

READING THE LANGUAGE OF THE BODY THROUGH BIOMARKERS

For those who are already familiar with the concept of cycle charting, it's most likely through some practice of Natural Family Planning; but NFP is actually just one thing you can *do* with cycle charting — the two are not synonymous. Cycle charting is simply the practice of collecting meaningful data about your cycles. NFP is when we interpret the data to answer the specific question: am I potentially fertile today? There are plenty of other questions we could ask when it comes to interpreting the data. Is it likely for my IBS to flare up today? Should I be expecting my period to start today? Should I be doing this particular type of athletic training today? These are things we can come to know about our body which generally relate to physical health and activity. But since humans are embodied souls, our physical state can impact the way we make decisions, how we interact with other people, and how we build virtue. We can therefore use information about the biological process of our cycle to help us understand: how can I communicate better with other people? How can I navigate my emotions more virtuously? How can I be more authentic in my interactions with other people and with God?

I return again and again in my prayer and in my work to one line from *Theology of the Body*: "The human body speaks a language of which it is not the author" (104:7).

As we gain more knowledge about this aspect of the *language of the body* — specifically, what our body is communicating to and through us throughout the menstrual cycle — our list of questions will only grow! Yet, the data that we need in order to answer any of those questions largely remains the same. So cycle charting may be used for NFP, or it may be used for management of certain health conditions or to guide our communication and relationships with others. Same data, different applications.

And what, exactly, is the data we can get with cycle charting? There are many different ways we can gain meaningful information about our cycles. I'm careful to say "meaningful" because there is a lot of information we could potentially collect about cyclical changes, but not all of it has research which helps us interpret what those observations actually *mean.* The current researched biomarkers for ovulation which we can learn to observe easily at home are: cervical fluid, basal body temperature, and urinary hormone metabolites. To a lesser degree we can observe physical cervical changes and even something called "mucus ferning," but because they don't have research which links them to the timing of specific hormonal events (yet), we'll skip over those biomarkers for now. Each of these things give us different information and can therefore be used in many different combinations to help women "read" what is going on in our bodies.

> *... cycle charting may be used for NFP, or it may be used for management of certain health conditions or to guide our communication and relationships with others.*

First, let's take a look at the primary biomarkers that common charting methods utilize:

Cervical Fluid

Cervical fluid is often called cervical *mucus,* because (nerd alert!) it is a non-Newtonian fluid that contains mucus molecules. But many women are more comfortable with the term *fluid* so that is what I, as an instructor and educator, tend to use. Cervical fluid is produced in the cervix, which is the lower neck of the uterus. If you imagine that your uterus is shaped sort of like a funnel, the cervix is the narrow bottom part which is shaped like a hollow cylinder. Inside the cervix are different crypts, which are recesses within which the cervical fluid is produced. You could en-

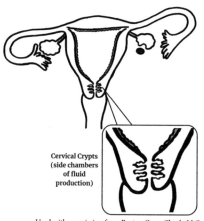

Cervical Crypts
(side chambers
of fluid
production)

Used with permission from Boston Cross Check, LLC

vision them as different side chambers within the cervix.

As we progress through our menstrual cycle, different hormones will act on these crypts and stimulate production of different types of fluid, which will flow beyond the cervix out into the vagina and then out of the vaginal opening so they can be observed externally. The sensation and appearance of this fluid can be categorized in various ways to help a woman understand where she is in her cycle relative to ovulation. In general, the pattern that women look for is a building up of "wet" or slippery fluid which has the look and feel of a raw egg white leading up to ovulation, and a drying up pattern which follows ovulation. Cervical fluid is a biomarker which primarily helps us track the presence of the hormone estrogen, which is a key indicator leading up to ovulation.

Basal Body Temperature

A woman's basal body temperature (BBT) is her lowest, natural temperature which is taken after a period of rest. BBT is a helpful biomarker because it responds to the presence of progesterone after ovulation. In general, women who track their BBT will learn to identify a set of low temperatures (prior to ovulation) to which she will compare her elevated temperatures (after ovulation).

Traditionally, BBT needed to be measured either orally or vaginally upon waking in the morning, before a woman has done anything which might impact her temperature (for example: taking a drink of water, getting up and walking around). In order to calculate a reliable temperature shift, the time at which the temperature must be taken had to be consistent within a cycle. For some calculations, it even had to be consistent across different cycles. This meant that a woman who had irregular sleep patterns, whether due to shift work or unpredictable toddler wakings, would not be able to use this biomarker reliably. Within the past few years, however, new wearable devices have come on the market which effectively eliminate the need for consistent waking times. These devices typically measure axillary temperature under the arm, or skin temperature on the wrist or finger. While research has yet to verify that these temperature patterns conform to the oral/vaginal patterns, many charting methods now offer support for users who choose this option.

Urinary Hormone Metabolites

Hormones don't just hang around in our body forever. Once they are produced and have performed their function, they are filtered, broken down, and eliminated. One of the ways our body does this is through urinary metabolites — in other words, hormones that have been broken down in different ways by our metabolism and are excreted through our urine. The presence of certain hormone metabolites within our urine can give us good information about which hormones are currently working in our bodies.

At the moment, there are three primary hormones we can test at home in order to gain meaningful cycle information related to ovulation: estrogen, luteinizing hormone (LH), and progesterone. Some of these tests use a simple dip-stick method which can be read by eye, or by snapping a photo and putting it into an interpretive app. Other tests require measuring by a specific device which will give you an interpretive reading, with or without giving you a quantitative reading of actual concentration levels in the urine.

The information you get from hormone testing varies based on which hormones you are looking for. Estrogen, as we have said, will give you indications leading up to ovulation. LH, as the pituitary hormone which is primarily responsible for inducing ovulation within the ovaries, is also likely to tell you about upcoming ovulation. Progesterone is a hormone which confirms ovulation.

CHARTING METHODS

By focusing on one or a combination of these biomarkers — in conjunction with bleeding patterns, which are often also considered a biomarker — women can begin to *read* the signs of various hormone activity within her cycle. Because each woman's cycle is unique and because each woman is unique in her lifestyle, preferences, goals, and circumstances, we cannot say that any one schema of observation or one combination of signs is going to work best for everyone. Fortunately, we have a great diversity of methods which allow us to take these three different biomarkers and observe them, chart them, and interpret them in different ways. This book contains an appendix which offers some more detailed explanations and commentary on what sort of person might be attracted to what sort of method. However, I do have some general advice if you're thinking about charting: pursue the route which allows you to achieve your goals!

Among NFP circles, we often speak about three different categories of methods based on the biomarker observations each one relies on. This delineation is imperfect, because some methods will actually offer flexibility that spans multiple categories, but it is useful for conceptualizing some of the basic differences among methods.

Cervical mucus methods, often called ovulation methods or mucus-only methods, use a single fertility indicator, cervical fluid. Common examples of these methods are the Creighton Model, the Billings Ovulation Method, and the Two Day Method.

Sympto-thermal methods use two indicators, cervical fluid and temperature. Common examples in the United States include Couple to Couple League, SymptoPro, and NFP International. Sensiplan is a German-developed method which has gained popularity in Europe and may eventually expand within the US.

Hormonal methods, sometimes referred to as "sympto-hormonal", may use a variety of indicators, but always have hormone monitoring as their distinctive feature. Common examples include the Marquette Model, Boston Cross Check, and FEMM.

All of these methods will function the same at a macro-level: you observe the signs of your method, record them according to the instructions given by your method, and interpret them to determine where you are relative to ovulation in the cycle. For couples who want to use this information for family planning, you also need to learn about how to identify a couple's "fertile window" — the time of the cycle when you would be able to conceive, which is also related to ovulation.

Yet even though the principles are the same, methods can vary not just in biomarkers, but also in the ways a method asks you to observe, record, and interpret those biomarkers. Some methods will have a 3-over-6 temperature rule to verify ovulation, whereas others will use a 4-over-6 temperature rule or even a mean temperature rule. Methods can have different instructions about whether you are supposed to wipe the surface of the skin in order to observe cervical fluid, or if you can simply observe the sensation you feel with fluid while walking around throughout the day. So, when I am consulting with a woman or a couple, I'm careful to not rule out a whole category of method too quickly. Someone who has a real aversion to checking fluid at the surface of the vaginal area can still be very successful with a mucus method, she just needs to learn the right one for her.

LEARNING TO CHART

The fact that so many methods exist can be a bit overwhelming for someone who is just starting on a journey to learn how to read this unique aspect of the language of her body. Having navigated many situations with "method switcher" clients I can also say that having so many options can be overwhelming for people who have tried one thing and are looking for something different, as well!

If you are looking to use this information for family planning, it is important that you work with a trained instructor. How effective a method can be — either at postponing pregnancy or at helping couples target their fertile window in order to try to conceive — is based on learning with a trained instructor who can check your comprehension and interpretation of charts. Charting is very straightforward — until it isn't. This is where you can benefit from the experience and training of an instructor. It used to be the case that instruction was offered locally and you may have been limited in method choice by the availability of certain providers in your area; however, it is now far simpler to conduct instruction remotely and the vast majority of teachers are happy to take clients online. Unless you feel very strongly about meeting with someone in person, you needn't feel like any particular method is inaccessible.

Once you've done a preliminary assessment of which methods you might be interested in, it's always best to meet with an instructor to check and see that you are a good fit together before making the commitment to learn with them. It is often more important to find an instructor you work well with and feel comfortable with than to try to identify the "perfect" method, because so much of your success with learning will be based on how well you and the instructor can communicate and can develop a relationship of mutual respect. There is always a balance, I find, between making sure that you're working within a system of charting which feels comfortable to you, and ensuring that you have the right person helping you learn and navigate that system.

If you are looking to use this information to help with a specific health issue, you may need to work with a healthcare professional directly. Not all NFP instructors have a healthcare background, and they should be upfront with you about the limitations of their training if you already know that you have specific health concerns or goals. Your options for methods may therefore be more limited, because some providers will have very specific charting methods that they expect you to follow in order to receive the best care. Whatever you give up in freedom to choose a method, however, will often be offset by improved results and a more streamlined approach to your overall healthcare.

If you are looking to use this information just to grow in self-knowledge and appreciation of your body, it is not necessary to hire an instructor or to work with a healthcare provider. You may simply want to pick up a book or join an online group and experiment with keeping track of different signs to see what your preferences are. If you find a charting method that you like, stick with it! If you are finding anything difficult or confusing to interpret on your own, then you could consider investing in an instructor to help you with those questions.

Regardless of which method you choose to start with, always remember that you still have options. I have a very wise instructor friend who likes to say to couples, "Remember: you are married to each other, not your method." The same sentiment applies even if you are not married: your practice of charting should be at the service of self-knowledge. If you just feel more confused by it, try something else.

There are actually two additional categories of NFP methods which don't include observation of biomarkers for ovulation. Because of this, their utility for some of the applications we will discuss over the next chapters is rather limited, but there are some situations in which this approach to cycle appreciation will provide you with all the utility and information you need.

Calendar-based methods use past cycle data and patterns without looking at particular biomarkers for ovulation within the cycle. The classic rhythm method falls into this category, as well as the more modern Standard Days Method (aka Cycle-Beads). Because these methods only work well for women in very particular cycle situations, their efficacy rates at postponing pregnancy are not as high as other methods; therefore, they are not very commonly used when other options are available. It's interesting to note, however, that some apps with predictive features are essentially calendar methods — so it isn't always the case that technology gives us the highest efficacy!

Lactational Amenorrhea (LAM): the suppression of fertility achieved by breastfeeding has been well-studied at this point. Women who meet very specific criteria for nursing frequency, bleeding patterns, and number of months postpartum may use LAM with a very high degree of efficacy for family planning. One of the functional benefits of LAM is that it does not require observation of biomarkers.

CAN I CHART WHILE TAKING CONTRACEPTIVES?

Let's address a very practical and common question: Whether a woman can effectively chart her cycles if she is taking synthetic hormones or has an IUD. When it comes to options for family planning, the Church has spoken clearly against use of anything which disrupts the natural function of the human body in order to "redesign" the effects of sexual intercourse. If a couple seeks to postpone pregnancy, the Church instead guides couples to prayerfully utilize Natural Family Planning instead. However, we also know that birth control methods are often prescribed by doctors to assist with management of various symptoms that are related to our menstrual cycle hormones, regardless of a woman's marital status.

For single women who are not sexually active, the biggest concern with contraceptives is the potential risk to your own health. It's always important to be informed about the pros and cons of any proposed medical treatment, and this area is no exception. However, for married couples who are sexually active, the concerns are a bit different and are worth briefly touching on here. For married couples, the guidance from the Church is that in some cases, health management can still be a permissible use for these tools through the principle of double effect. If an action has two foreseen consequences, one of which is good and the other is morally problematic, it may be possible to do this action with the intention of achieving the good effect as long as other important criteria are met. First, the action itself needs to be morally neutral, at a minimum. We can never intend for good effects to happen through evil actions. Additionally, we cannot intend for the good effect to happen as a direct result of the evil effect, either. And finally, there also must be an element of proportionality, meaning that the good (intended) effect must outweigh the seriousness of the evil (unintended) effect.

When it comes to the topic of birth control, the general consensus is that we could choose to utilize medical tools commonly called "birth control" to preserve or maintain serious elements of health — even if we know that it will also disrupt our natural cycles — as long as all of those criteria for double effect are met. While there are doctors who are trained to take a different approach to hormonal symptom management through restorative reproductive medicine, I know that these doctors can be prohibitively difficult to access and work with due to many different limitations. So, if the best option you have been given by your doctor is to utilize a type of "birth control" specifically for symptom relief, please know that this can be a legitimate application given the proper discernment. And if you have questions about mechanisms or moral considerations specific to the type of treatment plan you have been offered, please know that the National Catholic Bioethics center (ncbcenter.org) has a large repository of articles and summaries on this topic, as well as a consultation service which offers 24-hour hotline support.

But more to the point for the subject at hand: if you are considering learning how to chart your cycles, suppressing or altering our menstrual cycle function is really going to complicate things. Hormonal contraceptives work by overriding our natural hormonal fluctuations and replacing them with stronger synthetic hormones, either to mimic progesterone alone, or to mimic a combination of estrogen and progesterone. In most cases, the result of this is the suppression of ovulation altogether,[1] which means that you will not actually be cycling and therefore will not experience the cycle-related changes the following chapters will describe. Therefore, charting for ovulation while taking a hormonal contraceptive would not make sense; however, in many cases women who are taking synthetic hormones will still experience a bleed. This is not a real period, because ovulation is suppressed, but it is a type of anovulatory hormonal bleed which is still visible and is experienced much like a period. In these cases, we can cling to the fact that the dimension of *sign* is not completely eliminated: you can contemplate the goodness of how your body has created this endometrial lining, and the significance of your body's ability to create and shed this good blood.

If, however, you have been put on a copper IUD by your doctor, the story will be quite different. Copper IUDs work by creating inflammation in the reproductive organs in order to ensure that sperm and egg are unable to meet, or — in the case they do — implantation will not be able to happen. As one manufacturer explains, "It won't prevent your natural menstrual cycle. … [It] does not stop your ovaries from making an egg (ovulating) each month."[2] Because of the huge abortifacient potential, Catholic providers really should not be prescribing this option for women who are sexually active, and likewise — Catholic women who are sexually active should not be using it. But I have met with too many Catholic women who have been advised by their provider (who may or may not be Catholic) to use a copper IUD without being told about its unique mechanism. It begs the question of how well we, as a society, follow guidelines of informed consent prior to utilizing these technologies. But the point I want to make is that observing and tracking menstrual cycles is certainly possible with a non-hormonal IUD, because most women are still actually cycling. Women who are utilizing this device might have a more difficult time tracking cervical fluid due to the inflammation, but their cycle technically remains intact and they will therefore see many of the patterns that these next chapters will discuss. I have worked with some NFP clients who are able to successfully learn about and track their cycles for ovulation while they are waiting (sometimes months!) to have their IUD surgically removed. And because you can track ovulation, it is still possible to identify the potentially fertile window and abstain during that time to avoid the abortifacient action. So you can, technically, track your cycles in most cases with these devices. But just remember that they do interfere with certain observations and do not fall into the same moral category as other commonly prescribed contraceptives when it comes to symptom relief and medical treatment.

CHAPTER 10

Cycle-Syncing Our Prayer Life

Once you have begun to chart your cycle, a whole new set of information will be available to you, because you will now be able to identify which *phase* of the cycle you are currently in. At the beginning of this book, we saw an overview of the menstrual cycle that explained that ovulation — not a bleed — is the key event in a woman's cycle. Before ovulation, during the follicular phase, a woman's body is working hard to mature and release an egg, while sustaining a fertile environment. After ovulation, in the luteal phase, her body is then actively preparing for pregnancy, always hopeful that the egg that has been released will become fertilized, and new life will be created. These are two very different biophysical realities, and they are reflected in rapid hormonal changes. In addition to those two phases, which effectively revolve around the presence and function of the follicle in the ovary, we also can speak meaningfully of the menstrual phase, when all of the hormones "reset" and gear up to do the same process again.

Other than providing a neat and easy way to describe certain hormonal events, these phases mean that over the course of a few weeks, a woman's body will cycle through different energy levels and needs, depending on what processes it is focused on at the time. It therefore stands to reason that certain patterns may emerge in the life of women, related to the phases of our menstrual cycle. But what sort of things will we experience in the different phases?

Even without cycle charting, most women are familiar with various symptoms that are associated with our menstrual phase: In addition to the obvious experience of a bleed, many women feel some degree of cramping and fatigue as our bodies perform this important function. Also familiar are the symptoms of oft-maligned "PMS": premenstrual syndrome. PMS is usually marked by signs such as increased irritability, food cravings, and bloating due to water retention. To a certain extent, all of these changes are simply what you would expect from a body that is actively preparing for pregnancy. Our body wants to store energy, slow down, take on lots of additional water, and help a mother be more sensitive and attuned to her environment. However, these symptoms can become severe to the point where they interfere with our ability to function, and the diagnosis of PMS — or its more severe cousin, PMDD (premenstrual dysphoric disorder) — should be treated seriously and adequately.

In short, a lot of us are accustomed to the idea that there are certain times in our cycles when we don't feel great, and we tend to associate all of those negative experiences with the entire cycle itself. Unfortunately, many of us end up drawing the conclusion that our cycles themselves are the problem. But when we begin to chart our cycles and pay attention to the ways our moods and energy levels shift relative to cycle events other than bleeds, it's possible that mentality might shift a bit. When we internalize the fact that the natural changes our body goes through with cycles are fundamentally *good* and healthy rather than a *curse*, we can appreciate that there are easier times and more difficult times in our cycles, and we can start to think about *why* certain times may be more difficult. Symptoms are actually a form of communication that our body offers us. If I experience difficulties at one point in my cycle, I can ask: What is my body trying to tell me? And once we start asking those questions, we can formulate a deeper set of questions: Am I having difficulty because my symptoms are really that severe (and if, so, is that something I should seek help managing better)? Or am I having trouble functioning because my body is trying to tell me that I'm pushing myself to do certain things in the luteal phase that would be better to do in the follicular phase, or vice-versa?

In this latter set of questions we have thus encountered the concept of "cycle syncing," which invites us to consider what might be improved in our life if we were more attentive to the way our body naturally asks us to adapt our behavior. The term "cycle syncing" was popularized by Alisa Vitti in her book *WomanCode* in 2013 and has been taken up and applied in various arenas of women's lives since. In general, the concept of syncing with your cycle is to align our intentional body decisions — for example, what we eat, how we exercise — to reflect the changing physical and emotional needs our body cycles through in its different phases. The practice gained international press in 2019, when the US Women's National Soccer Team reported that they had used period tracking to help them train more effectively in advance of the World Cup (which, by the way, they won). Coaches and athletes realized that by taking the players' menstrual cycles into account with things like exercise, diet, and sleep schedules, they could improve performance and recovery time.

Before we dive in further, let's begin with a very brief overview of the key features that are naturally present at various times in our cycles. This isn't a perfect representation, because even within the phases we can meaningfully identify sub-phases such as early or late luteal phase. But this gives us a few general concepts to work with as we move further into discussion:

Menstrual Phase: Our bodies are breaking down and expelling uterine lining, which is hard physical work. Estrogen and progesterone are "resetting" to their lowest levels. Through bleeds, our bodies are eliminating key nutrients such as iron, which can lead to fatigue. Focusing on rest and renewal through our food/nutrient intake and activity level may ease symptoms associated with our periods. Symbolically, we are presented with a "new beginning," as we say goodbye to the previous cycle and welcome a new one.

Follicular Phase: Estrogen is increasing, along with testosterone. We may experience higher energy levels and improved mood, along with bursts of creativity, boldness, or determination. Our bodies may crave higher-energy exercise, and foods to support our

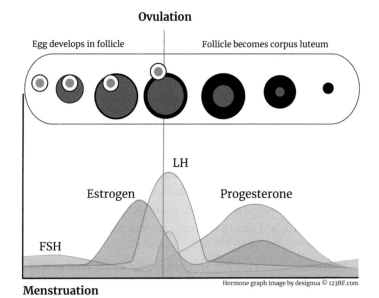

Hormone graph image by designua © 123RF.com

higher metabolism such as proteins, fibers, and leafy greens. Symbolically, our bodies are living out a particular type of hope — the desire to be fruitful and welcome life.

Ovulatory Phase: Estrogen is reaching its peak, and along with it comes an increase in confidence. Paired with slight physical changes that "improve" our appearance (e.g., redder lips, shifts in waist-to-hip ratio), our sex drive also increases as our body reaches its peak time of fertility. Nutrition can focus on foods that help us naturally clear any excess estrogen from the hormone surges, and we may notice our energy levels greatly increased. We may feel stronger emotional attachments to our husbands/boyfriends, or even a stronger drive to connect with friends and loved ones. Symbolically, this is the best time in our cycle for "fruitfulness."

Luteal Phase: Progesterone is now the dominant hormone, and the predominant drive is to bring "order" to our life. This is a time for handling administrative tasks that may have been dropped in the flurry of follicular and ovulatory energy. We need to be particularly mindful of stressors or sources of anxiety, as we naturally draw more inward and become more sensitive to our environment. We may notice lower energy levels, experience some physical changes as our bodies retain water, and have food cravings (especially sugars, due to slightly increased insulin resistance in our late luteal phase)! It is easier to be reflective in this phase, and in some ways we are forced to reflect on and confront issues that we have not paid attention to in previous parts of the cycle, so we may feel like it's a time when our "inner critic" makes a big appearance. Symbolically, this is the stage where we are "pregnant" with the anticipation of new life.

These general insights can be incredibly empowering for women, regardless of whether you are an elite athlete or a 9-to-5 employee who hardly ever gets a break from sitting at a desk. Respecting our cycles can help us be better versions of ourselves, because our well-being is tied into our unique cycle. Whether we are ovulating regularly or seldom ovulating, cycle charting can help us identify specific needs and strengths that our body is currently experiencing.

There are myriad websites, social media accounts, and even books that can introduce you to the concept of cycle syncing to maximize your workout routines, diet, or productivity levels. More research is needed to know how much benefit women could get from this sort of approach, and we must always be careful to not suggest that just because a person *could* do all of this work to cycle sync, there's some sort of moral imperative that she *should* do it. Yet there is some wisdom to be gained from the idea, even if we never implement it in our own lives. And so I would like to return to this quote from Pope John Paul II that has fueled so many of our reflections so far:

> What the different branches of science have to say on this subject is important and useful, provided that it is not limited to an exclusively bio-physiological interpretation of women and of motherhood. Such a "restricted" picture would go hand in hand with a materialistic concept of the human being and of the world. In such a case, what is truly essential would unfortunately be lost. (*Mulieris Dignitatem*, 18)

If Catholic women are to embrace this concept of cycle syncing, we must do so in a way that does not limit its applications merely to the physical needs of the body — and in this I would also include the emotional needs, which are so tied to our physical being. We know that humans are created as both physical and spiritual beings, so all of our amazing discoveries about the design and function of the human body should lead us to question: How can we integrate that knowledge with the whole person, body *and* soul?

Our Church has already offered some guidance in this area of "cycle syncing for the soul" in what we have previously explored as the cycle of the liturgy. This concept that the form of prayer and worship may remain largely the same, while the particulars meaningfully change, is something that we can apply to our own embodied experience of cycling as well.

It is common in the spiritual life to go through times of dryness, or to feel that previous habits of prayer that were so fruitful in one stage of life are no longer bringing us the peace and satisfaction they once did. To a large extent, this is normal. The *Catechism* speaks directly about dryness as "the moment of sheer faith clinging faithfully to Jesus in his agony and in his tomb" (2731). We may be familiar with the concept of great

This concept that the form of prayer and worship may remain largely the same, while the particulars meaningfully change, is something that we can apply to our own embodied experience of cycling as well.

spiritual darkness, exhibited by the likes of St. Teresa of Ávila, St. John of the Cross, or St. Teresa of Calcutta. St. Francis de Sales even speaks of it in his *Introduction to the Devout Life* as something we all tend to encounter: "Should it happen sometimes, my daughter, that you have no taste for or consolation in your meditation, I entreat you not to be troubled," he writes.[1]

As a woman living in the twenty-first century, with all of this access to new medical knowledge about the way our menstrual cycles affect energy and mood, there is now much more for us to explore on the subject of changing experiences with prayer. Perhaps it's not always spiritual dryness, but simply shifting levels of emotion, energy, and attentiveness, which may make some forms of prayer feel more difficult in certain parts of our cycle. I began to think about this because I noticed in my own life that there were times when certain types of prayer came easily — and I would think that I had finally progressed to a certain spiritual maturity.

Then just a couple of weeks later, those same prayers were difficult again, and I began to grow frustrated at some perceived failing on my part. Why was it so hard to form habits of prayer? And why, in particular, was it so hard to maintain them with facility and grace? These negative thoughts are incorrect for so many reasons, one of which is that I have often failed to acknowledge the reality that cyclical shifts in my body do carry spiritual effects. Would I be less prone to frustration and self-criticism in my prayer life if I embraced those changes?

By way of caveat, I have to say up front that I am in no way proposing that women who live by a particular rule — either as laid out in religious life, or taken up as a pious personal habit — should deviate from that rule in response to changes in her menstrual cycle. I am a Lay Dominican and know how important the fuel of a regular prayer life is for my vocation, and have experienced the benefits of this in my personal life. I do not intend to suggest that we should give up those necessary disciplines that unite us to a community, or to the wider Church. What I am about to propose, however, is an approach to devotional prayer that honors the unique virtues and efforts that are needed to sustain different components of your prayer life, at different points in your cycle. Knowing these things might help you develop an entirely new prayer routine, or gain meaningful insight into a beloved prayer routine that you already know.

PRAYING DIFFERENTLY WITH OUR CYCLE PHASES

In the description of cycle phases above, perhaps you were struck by immediate ideas about how certain prayers or habits could be a natural "fit" for different phases, and you are enthusiastically waiting to hear more. Undoubtedly, some readers may be tempted to abandon ship already, feeling that you don't experience these phases as described and therefore this whole concept is useless. I want to welcome either response here, as well as any degree of gradation in between. Our modern world offers us little opportunity to really "tune in" to these phases, so if you are not yet convinced that you experience these shifts, then perhaps your first step is not to try to implement a response to them just yet! Your first step is to start charting your cycle, if you haven't already, and invite God to help you feel more aware and comfortable with your body's changes. But I will also quickly return to the observation at the start of this chapter, which was that some women do not experience these shifts on a regular basis because they are not ovulating regularly. Or perhaps we can go deeper to acknowledge that certain medical conditions have a real impact on our hormones and our cycle function, which may obscure or even significantly change how our body experiences the different phases.

> *Cycle syncing our prayer life can be as simple as learning strategies to keep us from falling out of habits of prayer.*

I do not want any woman to feel that she cannot have a completely fruitful, life-giving, and grace-filled prayer life if she experiences irregular cycles. The simple fact is that God has formed you, and knows precisely how he wants you to love him and to be in relationship with him and his Church. Even more than that, God knows that humans weren't going to discover the hidden and intricate design of menstrual cycles for many millennia — so it would be ridiculous for me or anyone to assert that a woman needed to cycle sync her prayer life in order to be holy. My only intention right now is to invite us to consider this as just one aspect of the ever-unfolding mystery of how God has designed his beloved creatures to draw closer to himself.

Cycle syncing our prayer life can be as simple as learning strategies to keep us from falling out of habits of prayer. Have you ever had the experience of wanting to start a novena, and then petering out about three days in? I cannot count how many times I've done this, and always walk away feeling very weak and frustrated. At one point I was convinced that I just couldn't do novenas. But then I learned that it's natural for our resolve to fade when we are in the luteal phase. It's actually much easier for us to make and stick to a resolution in our follicular phase, when we have more energy to put into new projects.

What I took away from that one little insight is not that I shouldn't start a novena in my luteal phase. I should start a novena whenever I feel called to do so, but with the awareness that I might have to work harder to keep that resolution at certain times in my cycle. This is not a weakness, but an aspect of my biology that can help me understand why even certain spiritual practices come more easily at some times than others. Applying this one bit of information can also help us think about developing strategies for starting a new habit of prayer. If I would like to add a daily Angelus, it might behoove me to utilize the energy of my follicular phase as a sort of catalyst for embarking upon this new devotion.

This sort of approach to cycle syncing does nothing to alter the content or the rhythm of our prayer life itself, but just invites us to be aware of the way our cycle may affect our natural inclination toward prayer. It is a way that we, as Catholic women, can be intentional about bringing our whole self, body and soul, to our prayer life. Just by acknowledging the strengths of various cycle phases, we can perhaps better understand why we sometimes want to rush through that Rosary (hello, estrogen!) and why at other times we want to go more slowly. If you have experienced these sorts of shifting attitudes toward prayer, it might be worth charting that in line with your cycle phases to see where your particular strengths and challenges are!

Alternatively, we could intentionally pursue certain types of prayer or themes for contemplation in particular phases of the cycle. To a very small extent, I have come to do this in my own prayer life, because I have felt that I sometimes need grace in different areas at different points in my cycle, or different aspects of God resonate with me more strongly in certain phases. For example, I know that my ovulatory phase brings a lot of confidence and is a wonderful time for me to network with other people or reach out to form new relationships. But with that surge in confidence, I also notice a tendency toward pride, so I always have a copy of a Litany of Humility by my bedside for those nights when I am especially aware that I need this particular prayer. I will speak more about this relationship between our cycles and particular virtues in the next chapter, but first let's think about how we can turn to God in different ways throughout our cycles.

A very simple way to start would be to ask yourself the following questions in each phase:

- Where is it easiest for me to see God in my life right now?
- What qualities of God resonate most deeply with me right now?
- Where do I feel weak and in need of God's grace?
- What type of prayer "feels" right to me at this moment?
- In what way do I hear God drawing me closer to himself?
- Where am I aware of a distance between myself and God?

You might find that you do not notice a big difference in the answers to those questions throughout your cycle; in which case, creating a "cycle synced" prayer routine may not produce a huge benefit in your relationship with God, and it's probably best to put this idea aside. Any efforts we put forward in this area must always be at the service of an authentic relationship to God and his Church, so if they are not serving that purpose, then they are not actually helping!

But if you are finding some common themes and want to dive in more, here's a very brief outline of a sample prayer routine that links with the cycle phase descriptions offered above. Keep in mind that your relationship with God is unique, and some of these general suggestions may not be what God calls you to do, but at least this can provide an overview of the sorts of things to consider.

Menstrual Phase

Utilize lower-energy days for slower, more contemplative prayer. Prolonged prayer time may feel like too much, so go for shorter periods of Scripture reading, a Rosary, or another mid-length devotional prayer. Toward the end of your bleeding days, you may start to feel more energy and concentration. I have found that this is also a great time to go to confession, because we tend to feel more introspective compared with the follicular and ovulatory phases, but without the excessive negative self-talk that is common in the luteal phase.

Themes for contemplation might focus on the dignity of work, as your body works to clear out the uterine lining it has built up. You can also focus on Jesus' outpouring of blood on Good Friday. If you experience pain or discomfort, you can offer that up as your participation in Christ's salvific suffering, keeping always in mind that your Divine Physician does not desire this pain for you. You can contemplate the meaning of Sabbath and caring for yourself through rest in imitation of God.

A few Bible verses to consider:

Genesis 2:1–3: "Thus the heavens and the earth were finished, and all the host of them. And on the seventh day God finished his work which he had done, and he rested on the seventh day from all his work which he had done. So God blessed the seventh day and hallowed it, because on it God rested from all his work which he had done in creation."

Psalm 90:16–17: "Let your work be manifest to your servants,

/ and your glorious power to their children. / Let the favor of the Lord our God be upon us, / and establish the work of our hands upon us, / yes, establish the work of our hands."

Colossians 1:24–29: "Now I rejoice in my sufferings for your sake, and in my flesh I complete what is lacking in Christ's afflictions for the sake of his body, that is, the Church, of which I became a minister according to the divine office which was given to me for you, to make the word of God fully known, the mystery hidden for ages and generations but now made manifest to his saints. To them God chose to make known how great among the Gentiles are the riches of the glory of this mystery, which is Christ in you, the hope of glory. Him we proclaim, warning every man and teaching every man in all wisdom, that we may present every man mature in Christ. For this I toil, striving with all the energy which he mightily inspires within me."

Follicular Phase

Higher energy plus more tendencies toward creativity may mean that this phase is ripe for rich, extemporaneous prayer and for being intentional about making our work its own form of prayer. We may also find that it is easier to see the good qualities in ourselves, and we should be quick to thank God for those unique gifts that enable us to know, love, and serve him in a very personal way.

Related themes for contemplation could be the creativity of God, as we nurture our own projects in imitation of him. We can also think about fruitfulness, and what this means in our current state of life, focusing on the gifts that God has given us to pursue sainthood.

A few Bible verses to consider:

Psalm 139:14–15, 23–24: "I praise you, for I am fearfully and wonderfully made. / Wonderful are your works! / You know me right well; / my frame was not hidden from you, / when I was being made in secret, /intricately wrought in the depths of the earth / Search me, O God, and know my heart! / Try me and know my thoughts! / And see if there be any wicked way in me, / and lead me in the way everlasting!"

Matthew 25:14–30: This is the parable of the talents, which we need not quote at length here, but I offer the quick suggestion that it is right to meditate on our own talents and to consider how God has asked us to put them to use.

John 1:1–5: "In the beginning was the Word, and the Word was with God, and the Word was God. He was in the beginning with God. All things were made through him, and without him was not anything made that was made. In him was life, and the life was the light of men. The light shines in the darkness, and the darkness has not overcome it."

Ovulatory Phase

This is the time of our cycle when we are most seeking connection, so it might make sense to incorporate communal prayer into our cycles during this time. It will feel far more natural to pray with others in a group recitation of the Rosary, or perhaps to join a big group for praise and worship.

Perhaps not surprisingly, this is also a time when we may really resonate with the image of Christ as Bridegroom. The hormones in our bodies are oriented toward procreation and sexual connection, which itself is a mere sign of the deep communion we are promised with Christ in the New Jerusalem. If your heart longs for your heavenly Bridegroom during this time, then allow Christ to speak that love song to you! Know how deeply and personally God loves you, and make this a reflection in your prayer time.

A few Bible verses to consider:

Song of Solomon 2:10–13: "My beloved speaks and says to me: / 'Arise, my love, my dove, my fair one, / and come away; / for behold, the winter is past, / the rain is over and gone. / The flowers appear on the earth, / the time of pruning has come, / and the voice of the turtledove / is heard in our land.'"

1 John 4:7–12: "Beloved, let us love one another; for love is of God, and he who loves is born of God and knows God. He who does not love does not know God; for God is love. In this the love of God was made manifest among us, that God sent his only-begotten Son into the world, so that we might live through him. In this is love, not that we loved God but that he loved us and sent his Son to be the expiation for our sins. Beloved, if God so loved us, we also ought to love one another. No man has ever seen God; if we love one another, God abides in us and his love is perfected in us."

Revelation 19:6–8: "Then I heard what seemed to be the voice of a great multitude, like the sound of many waters and like the sound of mighty thunderpeals, crying, / 'Hallelujah! For the Lord our God the Almighty reigns. / Let us rejoice and exult and give him the glory, / for the marriage of the Lamb has come, / and his Bride has made herself ready; / it was granted her to be clothed with fine linen, bright and pure' — / for the fine linen is the righteous deeds of the saints."

Luteal Phase

This phase might actually see the most diversity in our prayer preferences, because women often report a great level of clarity and acuity in the days following ovulation, which then calms down as we approach the days leading up to our period. We may find, therefore, that some days are very good for prolonged periods of *Lectio Divina* or meditative prayer. Because we may also feel more emotional, it's possible that prayer periods may bring the gift of tears more easily during this time, or our mind may wander to more emotionally driven prayer topics. Whether and how deeply to yield to these promptings may require the work of a spiritual director, to ensure that we do not become too focused on producing "emotional fruits" during this time.

One theme to contemplate could be the way that our nesting

impulses during this time can lead us to desire order, in imitation of the God who brings order out of chaos. Since our bodies may feel a little worn down in the last few days of this phase, we can also think about the strengths that God provides in our human weakness. This is also an appropriate time for us to consider the biophysical way in which our body lives out *hope* during this time. Whether or not we are sexually active or trying to get pregnant, our body is programmed to operate as if the biologically-hoped-for event of pregnancy has already happened. How can we, as Christians, wait in this expectant hope, in this liminal area of the already-but-not-yet?

A few Bible verses to consider:

Genesis 1:1–5: "In the beginning God created the heavens and the earth. The earth was without form and void, and darkness was upon the face of the deep; and the Spirit of God was moving over the face of the waters.

"And God said, 'Let there be light'; and there was light. And saw that the light was good; and God separated the light from the darkness. God called the light Day, and the darkness he called Night. And there was evening and there was morning, one day."

John 11:35: "Jesus wept."

Romans 8:22–25: "We know that the whole creation has been groaning with labor pains together until now; and not only the creation, but we ourselves, who have the first fruits of the Spirit, groan inwardly as we wait for adoption as sons, the redemption of our bodies. For in this hope we were saved. Now hope that is seen is not hope. For who hopes for what he sees? But if we hope for what we do not see, we wait for it with patience."

CHAPTER 11

Cycles and Virtue

We've been speaking in this text about inviting Catholic women to embrace both the biological and spiritual dimension of their cycles, focusing on making sure that "woman" is understood in her human fullness as an embodied soul. We've explored how her menstrual cycle, as a biological function, operates in the dimension of sign and can invite us to consider how women uniquely image God. Yet there is an aspect of woman's *imago Dei* that still needs to be integrated with our understanding of biology, lest we fall into the error of thinking that women are completely controlled by our hormones. That element is our *will*. The *Catechism* states, "The human person participates in the light and power of the divine Spirit. By his reason, he is capable of understanding the order of things established by the Creator. By free will, he is capable of directing himself toward his true good. He finds his perfection 'in seeking and loving what is true and good'" (1704).

We cannot allow our conversations about the human person to forget that our rationality, which is expressed through our free will, is a guiding principle over the whole human person. It allows us to seek and to know the Good in everything of both the physical and spiritual world and to direct ourselves toward pursuing that Good. We see this echoed in the words of Christ: "'You shall love the Lord your God with all your heart, and with all your soul, and with all your mind.' This is the great and first commandment" (Mt 22:37–38). This tripartite command — to love with heart, soul, and *mind* — speaks of how important it is for us to not forget the rational part of our self, the part that allows us to freely love and enter into holiness.

We have already explored the ways we can use our minds to meditate on the meaning of our cycles and put that knowledge at the service of our prayer lives; but now I'd like to expand that conversation to propose how we might begin putting that knowledge at the service of our most basic vocation: the universal call to holiness, to become a saint. In addition to looking at our prayer lives, we must then ask how cycle charting could aid us in becoming more virtuous.

WHAT IS VIRTUE?

Quite simply, virtues are moral habits. Virtues are dispositions that allow us to reason rightly about a situation and to perform the proper moral action in that situation. A habit means something that we do without needing to pause and think about it. So, the cultivation of habits, specifically when we're speaking about the virtues, refers to the ability to respond and to do the correct moral thing in the situation, without needing to pause, consider, and deliberate in the moment, because we've already intentionally formed our will to act. When the situation arises where we need to exercise this habit, it comes almost as if by reflex or by instinct, and we do the right thing. While each of us may find that some virtues come to us more easily than others, the entire premise of virtue ethics is that the natural virtues are attainable by all — whether they are infused directly by God, or acquired through personal effort.

There are a lot of virtues we can and should practice, but they can all fall under the broader category of either the cardinal or theological virtues. The cardinal virtues are the moral virtues, or habits, that form the foundation, or the "hinge," from which all other moral virtues stem: prudence, justice, fortitude, and temperance. These are what we might call the "human" virtues, because they help us to live well with our fellow human beings, and to become our own best version of our human self. Every person is able to cultivate and acquire the cardinal virtues in order to live in right relationship with one another. The three theological virtues, on the other hand, are directed explicitly toward our relationship with God: faith, hope, and charity. They are not opposed to the cardinal virtues in any way, but go beyond them, because they have God, rather than other human beings, as their *object*.

Before we go on, I'd like to offer some quick definitions of the primary virtues, drawing primarily from Aquinas and the *Catechism*, to have as a reference point:

- **Prudence:** right reason, which helps us understand how we should act and to apply that knowledge to conduct our life rightly
- **Justice:** freely choosing to render what is due to another
- **Fortitude:** a firmness of mind that allows us to remain steady in doing what is difficult
- **Temperance:** to act moderately and rightly in the enjoyment of bodily pleasures

- **Faith:** to willfully assent to that which is True, especially concerning matters that are beyond our human comprehension
- **Hope:** the direction of the will toward a future that is decidedly difficult, but not impossible
- **Charity:** friendship with God, by which we choose to love God for his own sake and others out of love for God

The term "virtue" comes from the Latin term *virtus*, which actually means "manliness" — in the sense of being a perfect specimen of biological male human — a fact that has left not a few women puzzling over the years about whether this classical articulation of virtue is even meant to apply to women, or whether there might be such a thing as "men's virtues" and "women's virtues."

Yet because men and women are equally made in the image and likeness of God and are equally intended to share in eternal life with God, it does not make sense to suggest that men and women would somehow have different standards for moral perfection. The call to holiness and the beatific vision is universal. However, Catholic virtue ethicists must contend with a particular claim put forward by Thomas Aquinas: Despite the fact that men and women are both capable of receiving infused virtues equally from God, women have a harder time than men do in the natural acquisition of virtue.[1]

For Thomas, this is because women are more subject to their emotions, which means that it is harder for their reason to rightly order them to act in certain situations. Thus, the cultivation of virtue as moral habit is easier and more complete in men. On the surface, one could simply dismiss Aquinas' philosophy as the unfortunate product of Aristotle's view of women as "defective" men. However, as someone who spends many of her waking hours thinking about the ways in which our cycle phases impact so many aspects of women's lives, I have to admit that the fundamental conclusion — even if arrived at by an incorrect path — seems particularly intuitive to me.

If the entire concept of virtue ethics is that we need to practice virtues in order to acquire them, it makes intuitive sense that men might pursue a typically linear path to habit-building: *I practice this particular action in a repeated way, with increasing intensity or frequency, and thereby cultivate it as a moral habit.* This sort of approach is like planting a seed and watering it to make it grow. But for women, whose interior lives are built and fortified in a cyclical — instead of linear — pattern, that linear approach to cultivation of virtue will not be nearly as effective. What if, for women, the cultivation of good moral habits was less like planting and growing a seed and more like the formation of a river? What if the cultivation of virtue in a woman's life was a process of melting water carving its way through a landscape, all the while contending with the water cycle of evaporation, condensation, and precipitation that may, at times, run the river dry, and at other times cause the river to teem with rushing water? Over time, the river is carved into the landscape, and its shape becomes reinforced as more and more water runs through its channel with more and more ease.

> *But for women, whose interior lives are built and fortified in a cyclical — instead of linear — pattern, that linear approach to cultivation of virtue will not be nearly as effective.*

In a straightforward comparison, it may seem like the plant has the easier go of it. It's a much more straightforward process, and perhaps sees quicker results. But both the olive tree and the river give life to the people around them for centuries and are fruitful in their own unique ways.

To capture this in a specific example, let's talk about the virtue of chastity. Chastity is defined in the *Catechism* as "the successful integration of sexuality within the person and thus the inner unity of man in his bodily and spiritual being" (2337). Contrary to what we may have been taught as teenagers, chastity is not simply a virtue that keep us from having premarital sex. It is a virtue that, when cultivated, allows us to place our natural sexual desires (which are good, by the way!) at the service of our vocation and our pursuit of holiness as a whole person. In the context of a married couple trying to avoid or postpone pregnancy, this means that our sexual desires are placed lower in importance than some other compelling reason(s) why having a baby might not be prudent: whether that's something like maintaining the health of the woman, or being able to provide for the children we already have. So, tempering our desire to have sex with our spouse when we know that might lead to a pregnancy is a part of practicing mutual, or marital, chastity. I remember having a conversation with my husband once, during a fertile window when we were trying to postpone pregnancy, in which I expressed the thought that it wasn't particularly fair that I went through cycles with my hormones.

"Why not?" he asked.

"Because it means that there are naturally times when, to be honest, I'm not all that interested in sex. But there are other times when I'm SUPER interested in sex. And so I only get the opportunity to practice this more intense aspect of chastity for a short amount of time, whereas I think you have opportunities to practice it more often. So I feel like it's harder, in some ways, for me. And it takes more effort because when my libido spikes again after a few weeks of being lower, I sort of feel 'out of practice.'"

Of course, measuring the relative intensity of people's temptations isn't ever going to be accurate, fair, or productive. And I also understand that there's a reciprocity when it comes to sexual desire: When a woman is more eager for sexual intimacy, the man is usually more eager for sexual intimacy. That's kind of how the biology is built to work. But when I voiced this intuition, my husband agreed that it made at least a little bit of sense. It's a lot easier to create habits if we do them with consistency, and the fact that I didn't feel a consistent pattern of high-level sexual desire meant that I did not have consistent opportunities to "practice" integrating that into myself and our marriage relationship. On the surface, this slower and more gradual process of virtue building might appear as if women just don't have the capacity to build these virtues. But it actually just means that we need to build these virtues in different ways, employing different strategies than men.

Here is another way in which "woman" stands in as the archetype for all of humankind, in relationship to God. She naturally must view her progress in virtue as a cyclical affair, sometimes feeling like a vice or temptation has been conquered — only to realize that we have just not yet come around to it again. This approach to the natural acquisition of virtue calls to mind so many great spiritual writings that remind us, time and time again, that *conversion* is a constant turning back to God. In fact, the entire journey of the spiritual life is often less like a straight road, but more like a spiraling upward path that may seem at times to take us away from God, but is always leading us toward the apex at the center: "further up and further in," as C. S. Lewis says!

I am therefore going to propose some ways that women can begin to utilize the changing strengths and challenges throughout our menstrual cycles as a unique framework for virtue cultivation. We will speak of how certain virtues, or moral habits, may naturally occur more easily in some parts of our cycle, and how we can learn to identify and intentionally cultivate those habits in times when they come less easily. In this way, I hope to reconcile what seems like an internal inconsistency with Thomas' theories of virtue, by showing how the Angelic Doctor could perhaps have benefited from a little bit of twentieth-century menstrual cycle science.

BEGIN WITH CURIOSITY

A couple of years ago, at a presentation to a women's group, I shared some of my personal insights about what I like to call the "flavors of my personality" throughout my cycle. It's not that I'm actually a different person, or that I have a totally different personality from one phase to another, but rather that certain aspects of my personality come out more strongly sometimes than others. I spoke of the ways I was beginning to learn about my shifting patterns of virtue and vice, when one participant asked a very helpful question: "I've been tracking my cycles, using NFP for many years now," she said. "But all I know is how to identify when I'm probably fertile. How on earth do you start learning all of these other things? Where do you begin?"

In many ways, that single question has been the driving force behind this entire book, but it holds a special place in this chapter because she was essentially asking the question of how we can transition from a narrow and functional understanding of biological cycle knowledge — that is, understanding fertility — to a broader and richer understanding of the interplay between biology and our lived experience as women.

Unfortunately, there is no quick and easy answer to that question that is appropriate for every woman, because we all have very different and complicated relationships with our bodies. But one piece of advice can serve as the general starting point: begin with curiosity. We must give ourselves permission to see our cycles as fundamental to the shaping of our thoughts, emotions, and physical experiences, and to explore the unique way we — as whole persons — are influenced by these changes. Cycles cannot be seen as something in competition with our flourishing as human beings; rather, they are a constituent part of how God is asking us to live and work in the world. We should allow ourselves to at least be curious about this and to imagine how this could be a gift and a strength, rather than a weakness.

Curiosity in this area may lead us to begin the practice of a daily examen, by reflecting on the times and actions in the past day where we could detect the presence of God and reflecting on how we responded to that grace. Over time, this practice may reveal patterns in our behavior or even our ability to perceive God in different areas of our selves and relationships. When we begin to understand that certain virtues or habits come more naturally to us some weeks than others, we can then begin to make a plan for cultivating and exercising them throughout the cycle.

For example: You might find through intentional observation that you feel more naturally temperate in your dietary choices during your follicular phase. It may come naturally to gravitate toward foods that you know will do a good job of fueling your energy levels and nutrient needs, whatever those may be. But it may feel harder to make those choices in your luteal phase, because progesterone is making you a little bit insulin resistant, and therefore your body is naturally craving foods with higher sugar content. Your body isn't processing the sugars in the same way it had processed them a few weeks ago, so you suddenly feel like you're being tempted to eat an inordinate amount of brownies, which was not a temptation a few weeks ago. How many women have fallen prey to the notion that they are "breaking" a diet, or displaying some sort of moral weakness because they experience these varying degrees of cyclical "temptations"? Rather than becoming discouraged, this should hopefully give us a starting point for utilizing the many opportunities for change within our cycles to adapt varying strategies of virtue-building.

A QUICK ROAD MAP

Most of us — men and women alike — are not accustomed to charting out "growth in virtue" plans. Intentional growth in these areas is less about developing specific strategies and more about simply coming to an awareness that I am not quite as strong in certain virtues as I ought to be. Or perhaps I intuit a specific virtue would help me grow in holiness or in other areas of my life that I have identified as opportunities for improvement. Therefore, we don't need to develop a dense, highly detailed strategy for utilizing cycle knowledge to help us grow in virtue. Instead, what I would like to propose is simply a model whereby cyclical changes in our female bodies are taken into account as real factors when we do seek growth. I'd therefore like to suggest a basic sketch of what this might look like and allow you to reflect on this idea — and perhaps even try it for yourself.

> *First, do the work of identifying the places in your cycle where your moral strengths are more noticeable.*

First, do the work of identifying the places in your cycle where your moral strengths are more noticeable. It is likely not the case that one phase is demonstrably superior in all virtues, but rather that some virtues shine in some phases, whereas others come to the fore in a different phase. I'll give you a personal example related to humility.

Humility can be defined a number of ways, but the most helpful way I have found to think about it is "rightly understanding one's limits and strengths." This means that we do need to submit ourselves to our superiors, and especially to God. But it also means that we should be grateful for and willing to acknowledge the talents we have been given, so that we may know how to use them in service to others. As with all the virtues, humility strikes a middle road between a vice of excess and vice of deficiency. The excess vice related to humility is pride, where we think far too much of ourselves. The deficient vice related to humility is self-abasement or degradation, where we do not have a proper view of our own dignity.

What I have found through paying attention to my cycle is that humility comes easiest to me during my early follicular phase, when I have a clarity of mind that allows me to acknowledge both my gifts and my faults without too much emotional hand-wringing. During this time, it is possible for me to see myself as a creature who is very little, but who is also intimately and personally loved by my Creator. As I approach ovulation, however, that natural appreciation for my own gifts can quickly turn to pride and must be tempered by remembering my smallness. I start to swing toward excess and need to work harder at tempering my lofty opinion of self. But as I slide into the luteal phase I often find that I no longer focus on my gifts and instead hyper-focus on my failings, which means that I have to work to remember how much God loves me.

The cultivation of humility throughout my cycle requires self-knowledge and awareness, coupled with intentional exercises to maintain that healthy middle between two extremes that would both pull me away from humility at various times in my cycle. When I find that humility as such comes more naturally to me, I try to reinforce it. I try to seek out opportunities to practice humility, such as having conversations with colleagues who might elicit envy at other times in my cycle when I am less confident. Or I might take time to write out marketing emails when it's easier for me to see and communicate the strengths of my work without pretense or self-deprecation.

If we were following a linear pattern of virtue acquisition that expected a sort of baseline level of vice to either extreme of pride or self-loathing, we could see how this constant state of flux and adjustment might be perceived as a failure. We might conclude that building this virtue is just impossible! But instead, by being attentive to the natural ways in which our baselines shift as women, we are better equipped to weather the ebbs and flows of temptation.

Another example I like to think of is how the cycle of women means that our bodies are always in a state of "training" for a big physical event. Is it intemperate for a marathon runner to eat three large bowls of pasta the night before a race? No, instead we would say that the athlete is not intemperate in that moment, but is utilizing hard-won wisdom to know that carb-loading is prudent in this moment of intense preparation. The same runner would be both imprudent and intemperate if she routinely ate three large bowls of pasta every night for months leading up to the race. But when applied in a targeted way to her training, the occasional load is precisely what is called for. If we look the same way at the shifting needs of women throughout our cycles, we can apply a similar sort of wisdom. An action that might be considered lazy in one part of our cycle may be particularly prudent in another part of the cycle, and it takes a true "ascetic"[2] to be able to apply that wisdom rightly. For example, we may want to accuse ourselves of being lazy on our bleeding days, but prudence can help us understand that it is right to not fight our biology when our body needs more rest. And temperance can help us know what amount of rest is good and proper, without leading to overindulgence of physical comfort.

At the very beginning stages, we can therefore maximize our training by:

- taking note of times when particular virtues are naturally easier for us to exercise;
- seeking out times during those phases to intentionally practice and reinforce those virtues;
- being aware of how our practice of that virtue shifts as we change cycle phases;
- countering that shift to bring you back to the "middle."

In order to help you develop a working vocabulary for the things you might observe during your cycle, here is a very short list of some common virtues you may see shift with your hormonal "flavors" of personality, with their related vices of excess and deficiency:

Vice of Deficiency	Virtue (Mean)	Vice of Excess
Pride	Humility	Self-Abasement
Lust	Chastity	Frigidity
Cowardice	Courage/Fortitude	Rashness
Impatience/Impulsivity	Patience	Apathy
Gluttony	Temperance	Disregard for pleasure
Hastiness or folly	Prudence	Wavering in resolve, unable to act
Bad tempered	Friendliness	Excessive eagerness to please

FORMING YOUR COUNTERATTACK

Having begun to think about this idea of practicing and shaping the life of virtue in light of our cycles, hopefully you can see why I placed the chapter on prayer prior to the chapter on virtue. As Christians, we need to understand that our progress in holiness and virtue is not just about putting together a plan and having it go the way we want it to. There is a cosmic interplay between us as human beings, who strive for holiness through grace, prayer, and good moral habits, and the Enemy who would love to trip us up and have us become discouraged.

If we start trying to tap into our cycle phases in order to draw closer to God, you can bet that this will be met with spiritual resistance, and the Enemy will use the same practice to try to pull us further away from our Creator. That will become apparent when we see that just as each phase of the cycle comes with particular strengths, each phase also comes with particular weaknesses, and therefore each phase has areas where we might be particularly prone to spiritual attack. The Enemy may show up as our accuser, tempter, distractor, or the sower of discord — or whatever other tactic seems to break down the shifting chinks in our armor.

The *Catechism* tells us:

> Prayer is both a gift of grace and a determined response on our part. It always presupposes effort. The great figures of prayer of the Old Covenant before Christ, as well as the Mother of God, the saints, and he himself, all teach us this: *prayer is a battle.* Against whom? Against ourselves and against the wiles of the tempter who does all he can to turn man away from prayer, away from union with God. (2725, emphasis added)

In other words, we shouldn't expect that utilizing our knowledge of cycles to deepen our prayer life and aid us in the cultivation of virtue is going to automatically mean that prayer gets easier or virtues always develop more quickly. In some ways, we should expect that cycle syncing will mean that the battleground of prayer and morality becomes more specialized, requiring particular tactics and weapons. Of course, the sacraments and a firm resolve to persevere in prayer are the fundamentals, but your battle stance and strategy, not surprisingly, will need to be unique to you. What I offer here is just a brief introduction to some key areas cycling women may want to pay attention to, so you can bring those with you to prayer and, through the guidance and counsel of the Holy Spirit, launch a powerful counterattack. In this way, we seek to identify areas of temptation and weakness for what they are. It is a way of employing knowledge of our own biology to our advantage, rather than leaving it to the advantage of another.

Menstrual phase: When paying attention to the need your body shows for rest and attention, the enemy may try to accuse you of laziness or selfishness. If we have been trying to conceive, or our periods are particularly painful, we may be prone to accuse our body of "betraying" us because it is not behaving as we would like it to behave. We should counter these false accusations with prudence, temperance, and humility.

Follicular phase: As confidence increases, the enemy may increase your pride and tempt you to look down on others. You must guard against boastfulness, and use the strengths of friendliness to help you maintain a right relationship with others.

Ovulatory phase: The enemy may attack your sexuality, accusing you of lust, filling you with negative thoughts to discourage natural and healthy expressions of sexuality, or tempting you to unchaste actions. The virtue of chastity helps us to focus on the goodness of our sexual nature, in right relationship with all of our other activities, relationships, and duties.

Luteal phase: The enemy will fill you with self-doubt and cause your resolve to waver. You are prone to scrutiny and may be tempted to give up the good resolutions and challenges you set for yourself earlier in the cycle. You may accuse yourself of gluttony when those sugar cravings hit, and your anxiety may increase as you find it harder to fall asleep. Fortitude, temperance, and prudence — especially with regard to your bodily needs — are all helpful virtues here.

This concept of naming and shedding light on the tactics of the enemy is powerful for us to employ on our own, but is even more helpful when utilized in the presence of a trained spiritual director. Dan Burke, founder and president of the Avila Institute for Spiritual Formation, puts it thus: "Secrecy and isolation are among the most powerful tools of the enemy. … With all the floodlights on, the enemy's power is dramatically diminished, and he will often immediately flee. In this case, turning the lights on is the action of revealing a desolation, anxiety, or related temptation to either a good confessor or a spiritual person."[3]

CHAPTER 12

To a Deeper
Self-Knowledge and Love

Over the past few chapters, we've been exploring the question of how learning to chart our menstrual cycles could give us insight into various aspects of our inner female life, and provided a couple of unique ways we might utilize that knowledge to deepen our prayer and advance in virtue. But the act of charting and the information we get from charting can also simply help us appreciate certain aspects of ourselves as creatures who are beloved daughters of God. For some of us, this sort of reflection may come naturally because our own temperament, coupled with a relatively easy experience of cycles and periods, inclines us to a natural appreciation of them as reflective of good, healthy, biological function. But for others, we must admit that cycle charting forces us to face aspects of ourselves that we are not particularly comfortable with.

This could be because we experience painful periods, which make it hard to see how this could at all be good. Or maybe charting throws light on a medical issue that we were much more comfortable hiding under a bushel basket and trying to ignore. Many times, we also negatively link cycles and periods to our sexuality, which manifests as embarrassment or even shame about having a cycle at all — an unfortunate byproduct of education that never taught us to view our cycles as important in and of themselves, and only stressed the "dangers" of pregnancy and "unprotected" sex, whether from a religious moral perspective or not. Sometimes, charting cycles can even create an additional burden for couples who are trying to conceive — women may be tempted toward anger at their bodies if they see that their cycles aren't functioning optimally for fertility. These are all great challenges to a person's experience of charting that we must not be blind to.

In secular terms, knowledge is power. In religious terms, knowledge is love.

But I am always brought back to one key concept: In secular terms, knowledge is power. In religious terms, knowledge is love.

Cycle charting increases our knowledge about what is going on in our bodies, whether we like what we learn or not. Despite the fact that we cannot control the data we get from our various biomarkers, we can control what we do with that information and how it shapes our thoughts and actions. So with that in mind, let us now explore how we can both be empowered *and* grow in love of self and God through cycle charting. As our knowledge about our cycles increases, how can we learn to accept our bodies as they are (not as we want them to be!) and make the choice to love what God has made and called good (even if it's hard for us to see)?

CYCLE CHARTING HELPS US
EMBRACE OUR UNIQUENESS

Let's begin by talking about the obvious challenge that is present-ed when our cycles don't seem to be "regular." One of the most common objections I hear women make about Natural Fami-ly Planning is that they don't believe women with irregular cy-cles can utilize it. They don't believe that it's effective unless you have a perfect twenty-eight-day textbook cycle. Unfortunately, this misunderstanding is also incredibly pervasive in the medi-cal world. At my last OB appointment, my doctor reviewed my medical charts (not my NFP charts, unfortunately) and looked up at me over the top rims of his glasses. "And you're not taking any birth control, right?"

"No, I use Natural Family Planning. It's worked out really well, and my husband and I are happy with it."

"Ah. Well your cycles must be very regular then, so that's good."

I just rolled my eyes, because I have tried talking with this doctor in the past. I have tried explaining that his CDC chart that hangs on the back of the door lumps the rhythm method together with other, more effective methods of NFP, which is the only way they can get that incredibly inaccurate efficacy rate. I have tried explaining that while the rhythm method requires women to have a certain amount of cycle regularity, other NFP methods look for biomarkers related to ovulation and therefore are much more robust and flexible for women who don't have regular cycles. Apparently nothing of what I said before sank in, so in that particular moment I decided it was better to just get the appointment over with and move on.

I have used NFP postpartum when I didn't have regular cycles. And I have clients who have many different underlying conditions that make their cycles very irregular; even though we sometimes have to make modifications to protocols for them, they are still able to use NFP very effectively. Which means that they can also glean valuable information from their charts, even if they are only collecting that data for self-knowledge.

I would go so far as to suggest that cycle charting can be even more beneficial for women who have irregular cycles than for those whose cycles seem regular and predictable — first, because it provides incredibly valuable information about health that would otherwise go unknown. Cycle charts can reveal meaningful information about where ovulation is happening in any given cycle, how frequently a woman is ovulating, and how long the follicular and luteal phases are. Depending on which biomarkers a woman chooses to track and which method she is working with, cycle charting can also reveal helpful information about the relationships between hormones such as estrogen, LH, and progesterone, which is another valuable piece of data to have.

Second, it would be helpful for women with irregular cycles to chart because gaining true body literacy is not about trying to make every woman fit into a nice, neat set of expectations for her cycle. On the contrary, in order to use cycle knowledge to our advantage, we have to actually observe our own cyclical patterns and understand the unique way that our body undergoes and expresses this process.

For example: Because cycle charting includes observation of both bleeds *and* hormonal events related to ovulation, some women may make a surprising discovery when they chart. They may find that some of the bleeds they have been experiencing are not true periods, but are rather "anovulatory bleeds" — bleeds that have not been preceded by an ovulation event. We've already discussed previously how a true period must follow a complete cycle, because ovulation is the most important event. Without ovulation and the hormonal shifts that follow it, any bleed is considered some other type of hormonal bleed. It is not a period.

There are many hormonal reasons why women may experience vaginal bleeding that is not a period, and the presence of anovulatory bleeds themselves are not necessarily an indication that anything is wrong. They *do* mean that a woman who thought she was regularly cycling through follicular and luteal phases may not actually be doing so! This can be hugely empowering to discover, because it can also help us understand why we do or do not feel or experience certain things each time with our bleeds. A woman with PCOS (polycystic ovary syndrome), who may only be ovulating once every sixty-five days, will go through very long stretches of time in her follicular phase, even if it is punctuated by days of bleeding along the way. Despite the fact that the follicular phase tends to be higher-energy, with more positive moods for many women, women with PCOS tend to exhibit higher-than-normal levels of fatigue, especially in the follicular phase. We may not know the underlying mechanisms exactly, but in conjunction with insulin resistance (which tends to be common) and medication issues, we also know that the typical high ratio of estrogen to progesterone in PCOS can cause heavier bleeding and anemia. I have found that many of my clients with PCOS actually exhibit lower energy levels during the follicular phase and feel more energy once they have finally ovulated and are in the luteal phase. Will this be the case with everyone? No! But it does mean that knowing your body's unique signs is an important step in making sure that you are respecting and honoring *your* design and not comparing yourself to someone else's.

Another important example is not directly related to cycle irregularities, but has to do with how our brain chemistry and other bodily functions are intricately connected. Women with ADHD (attention deficit hyperactivity disorder) may experience higher levels of emotional dysregulation in their luteal phases, leading to a higher prevalence of PMS, or even PMDD. The theory is that because women with ADHD tend to have lower levels of dopamine receptors to begin with, symptoms are worsened in the luteal phase when dopamine levels in the prefrontal cortex are diminished, leading to a decrease in cognitive function related to emotional regulation.[1] While a certain degree of emotional dysregulation is present for many women as we approach our periods, ADHD-ers may find that it is even more pronounced. Women who experience these symptoms may want to speak with their doctors about increasing stimulant medication levels on premenstrual or early bleeding days, depending on where their symptoms tend to worsen. In addition, the premenstrual phase can be coupled with intense "brain fog" for women with ADHD, which could possibly be attributed to very low dopamine responses. All of this means that women with ADHD may feel like they have a very difficult time engaging in administrative or "ordering" tasks that tend to be a good fit in the luteal phase for neurotypical women. So, instead of pushing to fit the normative mode, women with ADHD may prefer to put "hyper-focused" activities in their follicular phase instead. This way of working with your unique body chemistry is not possible if women are never taught to chart and observe the various phases of their cycle in conjunction with other shifting elements of their moods and experiences.

CYCLE CHARTING CAN HELP US EMBRACE OUR OWN FINITUDE

To provide a really obvious understatement: Challenges with cycles and fertility are hard. Women who experience reproductive issues such as miscarriage, infertility, subfertility, or even "hyper-fertility"[2] — meaning that couples conceive easily even in situations when fertility is expected to be relatively low — face not only physical, but also highly emotional and spiritual difficulties. All of these situations challenge our concept of our "self," either because they eat away at our preconceived notions of feminine fruitfulness, or because we somehow feel like a victim of our own biology.

In many respects, this is a right and just response. It should be a disorienting experience whenever we are faced with the reality that the fallen world, and therefore our human experience of flourishing, is not as it should be. For thirty years we have known that women facing an infertility diagnosis experience equivalent psychological symptoms to those who have received a diagnosis of cancer.[3] It begs many questions about how the Church can and should respond pastorally to women and men who face these unique challenges. But it also reveals the lie that is offered by so-called "birth control."

When we make the effort to collect and interpret information about our cycles and fertility, one thing becomes readily apparent to any charter, regardless of their charting application: We are not in control. We have never been in control! The lie of the birth control industry is that we can switch our fertility on and off whenever we'd like. But how many women have gotten pregnant while using birth control? How many women have taken birth control for years, only to realize once they stop taking it that they are not able to conceive? The same goes for couples who have used NFP. There are certainly ways that we can improve or optimize the efficacy of a particular charting methodology, but the whole point of NFP is that our natural fertility status remains intact, whatever that happens to be. We can certainly try our best to keep our bodies healthy and work with our female biology to optimize our menstrual cycle health to make charts easier to interpret — but ultimately, we can't control this aspect of our biology any more than we can have absolute control over any other system.

I was recently chatting with an NFP instructor colleague who has been through some difficult experiences with cycle issues and infertility. She was reflecting on her past experiences, and one thing she said really resonated with me: "I am not in control and that I couldn't expect the chart to tell me something that wasn't true about my body. God was and is in control, and I needed to trust him despite what the chart told me."

When we allow ourselves to embrace our littleness as creatures, we advance in the virtue of humility, which Saint Thomas says "consists in keeping oneself within one's own bounds, not reaching out to things above one, but submitting to one's superior."[4] In this case, as ultimately in all cases, our "superior" is God. This is why the Church insists that couples who use NFP must allow their practice to be guided by discernment, and deference to the will of God, because issues will most certainly arise if we neglect humility and try to assert undue control over this aspect of life.

CYCLE CHARTING AS A PATH TO CYCLE APPRECIATION

One of the more interesting facets of my work over the past decade has been keeping track of attitude shifts toward menstrual cycles in both the Catholic and the secular spheres. Maybe cycle charting has not quite established itself as a mainstream practice, but I do see women from all sorts of different backgrounds speaking the same truth: Cycles are an important part of women's biology that deserve to be respected and understood. Related to this shift are changes in terminology, which I see trending away from "Natural Family Planning" toward phrases such as "Fertility Awareness Methods" or "Fertility Management Systems." But a different phrase is creeping its way in, specifically among Catholic circles, which is the phrase "Fertility Appreciation Method."

This phrase catches my attention because it acknowledges the meaningful distinction between simply being *aware* of something versus actually *appreciating*, or valuing, it. I may be very aware of the big hairy spiders that inhabit our backyard shed, but do I actually appreciate their value in the little ecosystem of that space? Do I appreciate how many other creepy crawlies are kept at bay by those spiders? No. I do not. Because all I see is the spider, and it makes me want to run away.

But here again we encounter the invitation to bridge that gap between knowledge and appreciation … and even perhaps love. Maybe if I invested more time and energy into learning about those spiders, that knowledge could lead me to a deeper appreciation of their role in the world and would eventually lead me to desire the good of a spider's existence. That is, in essence, what love is: to will the good of the other.

If you are one of the women who might think of your cycle more like you'd think of a spider — something gross and scary and perhaps something the world would be better without — then I invite you to consider whether this is an invitation to put learning at the service of love. It's very easy to fear things that we do not know or understand. It's very easy to get upset about things that seem like an intrusion in our otherwise comfortable existence. But spiders were lovingly conceived of and made by God. They reflect something of him. And if we, in our stubbornness and fear, refuse to see the goodness in the spider and to love it for the fact that God made it, then we are also refusing to see some aspect of God that only the spider can communicate.

Even if you generally have positive attitudes toward your cycles and periods, focusing on this concept of appreciation is also a way to improve your experience of cycle charting for fertility. I often encounter women and couples who have only ever been taught to think of cycle charting as a tool for family planning. This isn't necessarily a bad thing; utility for family planning is a very important aspect of charting. But it is very obvious to me when, during NFP instruction, that moment of appreciation just seems to "click." I especially love it when the man is the one who has the "aha!" moment. Occasionally, I'll be explaining the process of the menstrual cycle, and the information is completely new to him. His eyes light up, and it's as if he can see the woman and her feminine complexity in a whole new way. I love these moments, and I am delighted to witness them, because they make me think that I am witnessing a little resonance of Adam's original delight when he proclaims: "This at last is bone of my bones and flesh of my flesh" (Gn 2:23).

I understand that not every man has eyes to see in this way. And not every woman is going to see herself in this way. But I hope that by inviting men and women to at least acquire working knowledge of the menstrual cycle, we can create fertile soil in which the seeds of appreciation — and ultimately, love — will grow.

CYCLE CHARTING IS A TOOL AT THE SERVICE OF THE PERSON

As we come to the end of this chapter, I'd like to just take a step back to reiterate an important point: Cycle charting is simply a tool. As a tool, charting should have some sort of utility, whether that's for family planning or whether it's for managing our health, or perhaps you just find joy in the act of charting. But we must be careful that we never idolize the chart, or put undue pressure on the chart to be something it is not.

A chart cannot heal you. A chart cannot, in itself, diagnose you. A chart is just a visual way of representing data points. Many of my clients feel that charting can be a burden sometimes, and this sentiment isn't incorrect or wrong. This is why I'm very careful to say in my charting guides for teens and young women that if, at any point along the line, they're no longer feeling like there's a benefit to charting, and it's becoming a source of anxiety, they should never feel guilty about putting the practice aside. Charting does take significant effort, and we should be careful not to suggest otherwise.

Let's say, for example, that a woman is prone to anxiety, and she picks up cycle charting in order to track her anxiety along with her cycle phases. She is charting for health; but what if, at some point, she realizes that the act of collecting and interpreting data is actually increasing her anxiety symptoms? What if her anxiety finds a new way to manifest in and through her practice of cycle charting itself? This is a perfect example of when I might suggest to a single client that she take a break, and focus on her mental health instead. She could pick it up again any time she feels like the anxiety is under control, or if she finds that there is another application she'd like to use the charts for.

Even among my NFP clients, there are times when I suggest that they might want to put the charting aside! Couples who are trying to conceive may actually really enjoy the relative freedom of foregoing charting for a while. There is no requirement for couples to actively try to conceive by engaging in "fertility-focused intercourse." It's possible that there could be benefits if they chose to keep charting — like being able to give more accurate dating for ultrasounds and due dates — but couples can always return to cycle charting again if they haven't conceived within a certain amount of time.

> *At the end of the day, the only reasons you need to chart are the reasons that you give yourself.*

At the end of the day, the only reasons you need to chart are the reasons that you give yourself. I would venture to say that if I were not using my own chart for family planning, something like syncing my prayer life with my cycle or building virtue would, for me, not be a strong enough reason to keep charting. But because I am charting for family planning, I feel that my practice is improved if I am able to use the data in more ways than one.

Charting is a discipline, and it takes a fair amount of effort. So if we feel like the cost of charting is outweighing the benefits, then we should give ourselves permission to let it go.

Conversely, if charting starts to loom so large in our lives that it begins to eclipse other important things, it's worth taking a step back to make sure that we are maintaining balance. Christians must always work to love and respect the good things God has given us, without turning them into little idols. So do be aware that your charting does not become an obsession, or something that is undertaken over and against the more important realities of relationships, health, prayer, and the pursuit of holiness.

Additionally, we should always give ourselves permission to be imperfect charters — to let the perfect not be the enemy of the good. While it's true that achieving perfect method efficacy would require relatively perfect charting, we get to discern how much weight "the chart" has in our lives. Catholics talk a fair amount about "discerning" when it comes to big life decisions, and vocations, and family planning — it may seem like a daunting word. But really, discerning is simply about inviting God into the conversations you're having with yourself. It's a way to ask God: Is this practice drawing me closer to you? Is this helping me to see and experience the goodness of how you made me? Is this helping me learn more about myself, so that I can love you more fully? Is this bringing me closer to my spouse?

Sometimes the answers to these questions are painful, or even difficult to sort out. There's not a one-size-fits-all recommendation when it comes to charting, so the best thing we can do is to be honest and humble in making sure that this little tool of "charting" is rightly ordered within our lives, and is always placed at the service of God and the human person.

CHAPTER 13

Cycles and Community

Now that we've explored how knowing about our menstrual cycles can aid us in a deeper understanding of ourselves, let's consider how cycle knowledge can impact our relationships. Might our interpersonal relationships be improved by taking into account this aspect of a woman's interior life?

I remember many years ago speaking with a colleague who worked in youth ministry with me. She was suggesting that high school students should learn an NFP method, and I have to confess that my immediate reaction was to recoil against that suggestion. I didn't yet understand how fundamental the biology of cycle phases was to our physical and emotional well-being. It's not that I was concerned about them learning and then using that information to have premarital sex; studies have actually shown that learning about cycles in tandem with chastity education decreases sexual behavior among teen girls.[1] What I was actually concerned about was the mind of a teenage girl, and thinking back to my own temptation as a teen (and still as an adult!) to over-analyze things, especially about myself.

When I started charting my cycle as an engaged woman, it was a disorienting experience. I had gone from knowing virtually nothing about my fertility status, to having fertility be the first thing on my mind each day when I woke up and took my basal body temperature. I had been going through life for many years blissfully unaware that I might be ovulating or that my body might be feeling different because of which cycle phase I was in. Suddenly having all of that information — before I was prepared to act upon it for family planning — felt incredibly overwhelming and dissonant. I didn't want to be thinking about fertility so much before I was sexually active.

So, when my colleague suggested that teen girls should chart their cycles, my immediate reaction was the sense that asking teens to focus on fertility would be an incredible psychological burden. I worried that girls would be tempted to see every interaction with both female and male peers through the lens of their fertility status, which would be just another contributing factor to the anxiety and awkwardness of high school.

What I didn't understand at the time was that my own negative reaction to charting was due, in part, to the fact that I had been taught how to chart so relatively late in the game. I was in the throes of wedding planning, applying to graduate school, and going through some intense marriage preparation. It was not a great time to find out that there was a whole intimate side of myself that I had been completely ignorant of until two weeks previously. My whole worldview had shifted in the span of a few hours and, quite simply, it was a lot of information to try to absorb.

I see this phenomenon happen with some of my NFP clients as well. We sit down for an introductory session where I give them a "review" of the menstrual cycle and the biology of fertility, but it's clear that many of them never received this information in the first place. It's entirely new, and I can sometimes read looks of confusion, disbelief, or even total epiphany on their faces. At the core of all of these reactions is the realization that this knowledge somehow changes a lot of things. It doesn't change absolutely everything about a relationship, but it does change a lot. Does it change things for the better?

My previous worry with teens was that unless a person was ready to implement this knowledge in a constructive way with family planning, the shift could only be detrimental. But this was still rooted in the misunderstanding that cycle charting was exclusively about fertility — and hopefully at this point in our text, I have successfully made the case that it is not. We've already seen how basic cycle

> *How can basic cycle knowledge be used to draw us closer to the people around us?*

knowledge can be used to help us draw closer to God, and to better understand and love ourselves as unique and unrepeatable images of our Creator. Now we can apply that same sort of thought process to this question: How can basic cycle knowledge be used to draw us closer to the people around us? How can we use that fundamental relationship with God to improve our relationships with our brothers and sisters?

CREATING A CULTURE OF CARE

At a minimum, I'd like to put forward the idea that simply knowing about the various ways a woman's body needs care throughout her cycle is a wonderful way to care for one another better. In terms of friendships, this has immediate applications for a girl as soon as she or a friend experiences her first period bleed. Middle school is a notorious time for girls' peer relationships, in part because their bodies are influenced by hormone fluctuations that are new and potentially disruptive to their friend groups. Tensions may arise that were never present before.

To a certain extent, we should accept this as a normal part of adolescent development. Pre-teen brains are different. Their bodies are becoming different. It's a part of growing up that our interests diverge and our friend groups shift. But there are also aspects of peer relationships between girls that could be preserved and better nurtured if girls were more aware of caring for their own cyclical bodies, and extending that same care to their friends.

If we fast-forward to young adulthood, I imagine that many of us have had the experience of pushing ourselves to do something with a group of friends when our bodies really just wanted us to rest. I've had clients share stories with me about all those times they ended up going out to the dance club, despite feeling really low energy. Or they went on a long hike because they didn't want to disappoint a friend. But in all of those cases there was a common thread: They went along with high-energy plans, despite knowing that their body was craving rest, and had an awful time. It wasn't a great night or day out with friends — they were grumpy and just wanted to go home.

On the flip side, we've also all experienced friends who mysteriously cancel plans with little or no satisfactory explanation. Depending on your personality type, you may naturally take this in stride, or you may feel really hurt by these actions. This was a situation that a mother wrote to me about what her middle school daughter was experiencing:

> My daughter and I did your Cycle Prep course, and a few days after that she was expecting to go on a hiking trip with one of her best friends. They had been planning this for a long time, but the morning of the hike, her friend called and said she didn't feel up to hiking. She

canceled, and I just knew that my daughter was crushed. Before Cycle Prep, she probably would have gotten really angry at this friend and been in quite the mood all day. But instead she said something that surprised me: "Mom, I wonder if my friend is on her period or maybe in her luteal phase. Maybe her body is telling her that she needs to rest instead of going on this hike. I'd still like to hang out with her. Do you think we could call her back and invite her to watch a movie instead?"

Sure enough, we called back and the friend was happy to switch plans. The girls had a great time, all because my daughter was aware enough to think that something was going on physically, rather than assuming that the girl just didn't want to spend time with her.

Can you imagine the "girl drama" that could be avoided if we all were intentional about creating this sort of space for one another? Or how our relationships with male friends might be enriched if they were simply aware that women sometimes needed this sort of accommodation?

This is what I call in my programs the commission to build a "Culture of Care" for one another with cycle knowledge. It's a simple way that we can bring female biology into our awareness of "togetherness," by simply respecting and responding to the other person's needs. Of course, the corollary of this is that women and girls need to feel that they are empowered to communicate those needs and to expect that those needs will be heard, which can be a difficult thing if we are taught that cycles are somehow an inherently shameful topic to bring up. So building this culture of care means that we need to:

- teach all people about menstrual cycles and the shifting needs of women's bodies while cycling;

- teach girls and women how to observe the cues their bodies give them;
- teach girls and women how to generously respond to those cues to nurture their bodies;
- encourage girls and women to communicate those needs to close people in their lives; and
- make sure that all people extend care and respect to one another when needs are expressly communicated, or be attuned to times when they are implied.

If we do this, we will have built up a community where women's cyclical biology is welcomed as part of the social dynamic, which allows us to create relationships that are adaptable and responsive to shifting interplay between friends.

Imagine also how our conversations could be better, or the experience of women in the Church could be better, if we were all more educated on the complexities of the menstrual cycle and fertility. Insensitive comments about family size, made simply out of ignorance, could be avoided with a better communal understanding of reproductive biology. Snide comments about women's "fickleness" wouldn't make sense if more people appreciated the various strengths and challenges women undergo with their shifting hormones.

Cycles need not be the central topic of conversation among friends — they need not ever be mentioned explicitly, if that's the preference — as long as the cycle awareness of all parties is present, and the mutual respect is therefore undergirding the relationship.[2]

WOMEN'S COMMUNITY
Nothing quite drives home the point that people were created to live and serve in community than the experience of being an isolated, postpartum new mom. When my first baby girl was born,

my husband and I had barely been married for a year. We got married, moved to a new city, started graduate programs, and had just a few weeks to try to make friends before I got pregnant and began suffering from hyperemesis gravidarum. The severe exhaustion, dehydration, and starvation that accompanied my constant vomiting made it impossible for us to forge any new relationships. We were literally in survival mode, which meant that a few weeks after our new baby was born and our amazing mothers had gone back to their respective homes, we were very much alone.

This was back in the heyday of the "Catholic mom blog," so I found myself trying desperately to form a sense of community from my living room couch by devouring and occasionally responding to blog posts from women I quickly began to think of as friends — despite the fact that they had no idea who I was. I was trying to find someone who understood and could explain more about the physical and emotional experiences I was undergoing as a new mom. Why had I never heard about postpartum night sweats? Why did no one tell me that breastfeeding was hard? Or that afterbirth pains could leave you begging for an epidural all over again?

It was such a relief to know that even if the connection was virtual, I was not alone in these struggles and these questions. And this is also why I am never surprised when a woman comes to me for NFP instruction and then ends up calling me after a harrowing OB-GYN appointment, because I am literally the only person in her life besides her husband to whom she can talk about her cycles. Despite having very loving mothers, and even sometimes a bunch of sisters, it's not uncommon for my clients to feel that they are very much alone in their experience of cycles and periods. Yet there is always an undercurrent in their stories that affirms, "It's not supposed to be this way. We should be able to have a community to share this with."

This desire reflects the need for a different sort of community than what is described in my postpartum experience above — a community in which women freely share their experiences and their cyclical life with one another, in order to pass along wisdom and to know that even though their lived experience is unique, they are not alone. This was the same ache that Adam felt in the Garden of Eden, as he experienced the pangs of original solitude; this is the same impulse that senses how the human *imago Dei* is deepened through our experience of communion with others. It manifests in a particular physical way through male-female relationships in marriage, but it can still be felt deeply at any point we realize that we hunger for an "other" to be with us. And as much as we delight in the companionship of men, whether in marriage or in friendship, we have to acknowledge that other women can be "with us" in our experience of cycles and periods in ways that men, or even our children, cannot.

My simple suggestion is for Catholic women to not apologize for wanting to speak about their female bodies.

This is the sort of community that some modern feminists are trying to create by forming "Red Tent" gatherings, based on Anita Diamant's novel of the same name. There is a hunger for contemporary women to have a space like a menstrual hut, where they can gather with other women to share stories and be affirmed in their cyclical bodies. Other groups like this are growing in order to create intentional spaces for girls to have a ceremonial welcome into "womanhood" upon menarche.

Can Catholic women find a resonance of their own good desires in these communal events? Despite the particulars of some of these programs, which may sometimes be at odds with our understanding of human sexuality and the dignity of the body, there is something we can learn from this contemporary impulse to build communities where women welcome other women into the art of living as a woman. Likewise, there is much that could also be written about intentional community experiences for men. So, how can we be proactive about meeting this desire for communion and openness, without feeling like we teeter on the verge of worshiping our bodies, or overemphasizing our female bodies over and against men or the health of our souls?

My simple suggestion is for Catholic women to not apologize for wanting to speak about their female bodies. I have seen so many times when women, in the context of a women's book club or prayer group, will shy away from openly sharing their thoughts about how aspects of our faith resonate with or challenge our embodied experiences as women. I have also witnessed the beautiful fruits of women's conversations when those topics are openly welcomed, in an atmosphere of faith seeking understanding about the meaning of our bodies. It's okay to wrestle with the feeling that certain theologians articulate theories about the Blessed Virgin Mary that make us uncomfortable with our bodies. It's okay to share about the fact that excessive period pain makes it difficult to focus on prayers, or to get to Mass. It's more than okay for us to share about the struggles of lust and the shame we may feel when our libido is going crazy during ovulation. We need to hear more voices of faithful Catholic women who are genuinely seeking holiness in the middle of these experiences, so that we can build collective wisdom that will inform the Church in the future.

We also need the holy friendships of other women who will help us feel that we are not alone and will help us process our femininity through the lens of the Gospel. I will never forget the day when, as a postgraduate Campus Ministry intern, I was approached by an undergraduate woman who was in the liturgical choir I served. In addition to singing with the choir and being a part of the leadership team for liturgical music planning, it was my role to provide a brief reflection as part of our weekly prayer. About two months into the school year, this young woman pulled me aside and thanked me, just for being a "strong feminine voice of faith." She explained that the previous intern, who was male, was also wonderful, and she truly enjoyed his reflections. "You reflect on a lot of similar things," she explained, "but you somehow do it differently. It makes me appreciate how God's voice can speak differently in and through women, which is something I hadn't really thought of before."

Nothing about that particular incident was related to menstrual cycles or periods. But it has stuck with me through the years as I ponder the various ways female voices speak to one another about God. And it reaffirms my deep sense that women's voices are not only needed in the preaching of the Gospel through our daily lives — we are needed in the articulation of our embodied female experience. This goes for everything I have been saying about reflecting together as Catholic women, but also in the very important aspect of just handing down wisdom about cycle health. It surprises me how little my clients know about their mothers' cycle history. "I know she had to have a hysterectomy well before menopause," one client said, "but I don't know what for. And I really don't know how to ask. I wonder if she also had endometriosis like I do."

These are easy fixes! At least they are easy in theory. All we have to do is give ourselves permission to ask questions — or better yet, to willingly share our own experiences, questions, and knowledge when it's appropriate to do so. All NFP teachers would probably agree that even in everyday conversations, people will be a lot more open and honest with us about very personal things, because they need a space to talk about it, and they know that we are a "safe space." So my invitation for all women is not that we need to be aggressive over-sharers with our personal gynecological history, but simply to let our friends know through our actions and through the things we share, that we are a "safe space" for these conversations and that they are not alone.

WOMEN'S RELIGIOUS COMMUNITIES

Before closing this chapter on cycles and community, we now have to come to a topic that always piques the interest of Catholics when I talk about cycle charting: women's religious communities. After all, God doesn't just shut off a woman's menstrual cycle the minute she makes perpetual vows. And unlike most married women who will be pregnant at some point in their lives, a religious sister or nun will likely have no interruption in her cyclical patterns until she reaches menopause. So she will have even *more* cycles than the rest of us!

When it comes to cycle charting, specifically, I have spoken with many religious sisters who have told me that there are unique barriers to acquiring this knowledge and instituting this practice in their communities. At some point, a book needs to be written about the specific challenges women religious face when it comes to gynecological health. It would explore the dynamics of communities where the male spiritual director or religious superior directly prohibits cycle charting educational opportunities, or when a large number of sisters struggle with the goodness of their bodies because they were raised within purity culture or in a home where sexuality was considered inherently shameful and sinful. It would talk about the higher prevalence of ovarian cancer among these populations,[3] leading to some interesting questions about why we aren't investing in cycle charting for all religious women in order to facilitate earlier detection of such cancers. Let's write that book.

But for now, what we will focus on is this concept of cyclical interpersonal dynamics when you live in close quarters with lots and lots of other women. What difference does it make when this notion of the "Culture of Care" is tied up not just in friendships, but in the relationships between women who may or may not particularly *like* one another — but are all committed to loving, praying, working, and serving together nonetheless?

We might think that this is like the dynamics in a nuclear family that happens to have a lot of girls, but it's actually quite different, because a religious community is able to pick and choose its members. Women discern their individual vocation with particular communities, but the community also discerns whether it feels called to accept and admit those individuals. And it is completely within the purview of a women's religious community to take into account what they know about the physical health of inquirers, to discern whether their community is willing and equipped to pick up and carry this particular cross.

In some cases, this means that religious communities knowingly admit women who have severe menstrual symptoms. In particular, I know of a very small community that is bending over backward to accommodate a young novice with crippling period pain and endometriosis. They want to care for her and are seeking medical expertise, but they also know that there are times when this young sister is simply incapable of engaging in their community apostolate. They might plan to have her assisting with elements of a youth retreat, only to find that she must remain in bed that day and the other few sisters are required to fill in. At least for now, the sisters are saying "yes" to this aspect of their mutual vocation, which is a beautiful, challenging — and some may say very impractical — step to take, but other communities may discern differently. This is therefore a very different sort of dynamic than a relationship between friends.

On a very practical level, cycle charting can help communities like this, because it gives them a window into health issues that their sisters may be experiencing. We mustn't forget that cycles are considered a vital sign for girls' and women's health, and in many ways the spiritual health of a religious community is tied to the sisters' ability to care for the physical health of its members. Cycle charting can thus be considered a very practical way for women's communities to have a better sense of the overall physical health of their community and respond more quickly and directly when heath issues manifest on cycle charts. Quicker diagnosis and treatment can lead to less financial burden on the community as a whole, and fewer sisters languishing as they wait for answers. I have seen that play out in my own life, as a woman who has suffered from migraines of varying intensity and frequency over the years. Neurologists assume that migraines in women are usually hormonal, and I would have needed to wait three to six cycles on a particular medication to exclude that assumption if I hadn't already been equipped to show my doctor that my migraines did not track with my cycle phases. His comment at the time was, "Well, that just saved us a lot of time and money. That's neat."

Yet even without irregular cycle or menstrual disorders at play, knowing about cycles could contribute something positive to community life. At first glance, it seems that certain religious communities are some of the least likely places to be able to adapt to shifting cyclical needs. Strict prayer schedules and routines are some of the real blessings of religious life, allowing members to work and pray together within a relatively predictable daily rhythm. Communal meals do not easily accommodate some of the dietary needs our bodies have at different points in the cycle. And large community projects need to happen regardless of whether we are naturally inclined to those tasks or not.

This is where the concept of virtue-building with our cycles can truly come in handy, and strategies for working with our cycles even amidst regular prayer routines can be a benefit. When we understand and cooperate with our natural biology rather than feeling like we need to fight against it, many aspects of communal living can be more easily managed — this applies to both family life and religious life. It allows us to develop proactive strategies to navigate our own strengths and weaknesses, rather than always being "reactive" in our responses.

For example, let's imagine that there are two sisters who don't love each other's company, but they do try hard to love each other and get along. Sister Kateri, in particular, has never been fond of Sister Josephine. Sometimes this amounts to a tiny annoyance that she offers up during times when they are expected to work in the kitchen together. But other times, for reasons Sister Kateri just cannot understand, Sister Josephine gets on every last inch of her nerves, and she truly has to fight the urge to snap at every little thing Sister Josephine does.

Now imagine that Sister Kateri has learned through cycle charting that her temper flares in the few days before her period. She sees that she is next scheduled to work with Sister Josephine in the kitchen smack dab at the end of her luteal phase, when she is likely to be more irritable. This need not occupy an inordinate amount of mental space, because after a certain amount of time the self-knowledge gained with cycle charting becomes like background noise — something we take for granted. But because she knows this about herself, Sister Kateri can be proactive before her next stint in the kitchen with Sister Josephine, by offering up extra prayers for harmony between them and also paying a little bit more attention to fortifying her mental state. It may even help her to simply acknowledge that anger is a general challenge for her during this time in her cycle, so she works very hard to avoid making her frustrations personal and taking them out directly on Sister Josephine, as she has sometimes done in the past. Of course this same sort of approach could be applied in the workplace or at school, but religious sisters not only work together — they live together, pray together, and share in the same communal vocation. Thus it becomes even more important for those interpersonal relationships to be nurtured and intentionally cultivated.

Perhaps you may object that this basic level of self-knowledge is already a part of women's everyday lives; after all, many of us are able to recognize emotional or behavioral patterns that line up relatively closely with our period. But without knowing exactly where ovulation is on our cycle, at best we're utilizing a sort of "rhythm method" approach. What if Sister Kateri has PCOS and has a high variability in cycle lengths? Or what if she doesn't experience irritability where we might expect it in the luteal phase, but instead she gets extra cranky and stressed in the few days before ovulation?

Sisters who thus understand how their biological states contribute to interpersonal dynamics have the opportunity to create a community life that is more acknowledging of and receptive to these uniquely feminine aspects of their vocation. I hope that religious women can more easily see the beauty of their witness as brides of Christ, embodying the liturgical cycles of our Mother Church in both the order of nature and in the order of grace.

CHAPTER 14

Cycles, Marriage, and Family Life

For the vast majority of my current clients, cycle charting was a skill first learned in the context of marriage and family planning. Lower divorce rates are often cited, along with increased communication and sexual satisfaction among NFP users compared with nonusers[1] — but statistics do not tell the whole story. Only God can tell the whole story of how a couple receives, responds to, and overcomes obstacles to his grace in the sacrament of marriage, especially through their sexual relationship. So this chapter is not going to attempt to unpack all of those dynamics; instead, we will take a quick look at some ways that a woman's cyclical changes can impact a couple's experience of charting for NFP and then take it a step further to inquire about how married life can be enriched when husband and wife are both aware and appreciative of this aspect of female biology.

NATURAL FAMILY PLANNING

In *Humanae Vitae*, Pope Paul VI says that in order to practice responsible and generous parenthood, husband and wife should have an awareness of and respect for the biological processes involved in procreation. In other words, we should know how sex works, and we should honor that natural design. When it comes to family planning, then, couples who discern a serious need to postpone pregnancy are able to utilize knowledge of natural rhythms of fertility and infertility in order to avoid intercourse during the fertile time. This is called Natural Family Planning.

I remember giving an NFP presentation at a marriage preparation retreat once, very soon after I had become an instructor. The tension in the room was palpable: This was not a group of people who were well-disposed toward the idea of NFP, and I am sure I stumbled awkwardly through various elements of the presentation. At the end, I asked if anyone had any questions, and immediately a hand shot up in the middle of the room. It belonged to a woman who didn't actually have a question. She hardly waited for me to point in her direction before barking out, "I've noticed you only talked about a woman observing her signs of fertility. Seems to me this is a huge step backward for women's equality — making her put in all the work." Yikes. I probably looked like a deer in headlights, and I remember my heart racing as my palms got sweaty. Dealing gracefully with aggressive confrontation is not really my forte. What I managed to say was something like this:

Natural Family Planning does rely heavily on tracking data observed from a woman's biomarkers. That is true. And it is also true that it requires effort to observe, track, and interpret those biomarkers. But the reason we focus on a woman's cycle is not because the Church thinks that women are somehow "responsible" for fertility; it's because a woman's menstrual cycle is precisely the thing that makes NFP work! If women were designed like men, we would be potentially fertile all the time, and couples who wanted to avoid pregnancy would have no natural option for doing so. The fact that a woman goes through periods of fertility and infertility means that the couple actually has an opportunity to utilize those rhythms together. Couples need to understand that, strictly speaking, neither of them is fertile on their own. Fertility is a shared concept and shared reality, so responsible and generous spouses must ensure that family planning related to fertility is also a shared endeavor. And so part of learning how to chart with NFP is helping a couple learn to track and interpret data together, and to take mutual responsibility for actions based on their shared fertility. That doesn't make it easy. And it doesn't mean that it will always look equal in terms of effort required to get the data. But I tell my client couples that if, at any point, the woman feels like she is shouldering this burden alone, they are doing it wrong and something needs to change.

Now that I have been an instructor for over a decade, I can honestly tell you that for some of my clients, that woman's concerns seem really valid. We aren't doing a service to the Church if we insist that every couple who practices NFP is automatically insulated from these sorts of imbalances in a relationship. So, the first aspect of charting for NFP that needs to be addressed is the practical question: How do couples actually keep charts, *together?*

In my own practice with clients, I am careful not to tell them that cycle charting together needs to look a certain way. I have seen enough couples to know that what works for one marriage is not going to work for another. But in all marriages, it is important for the woman to not feel that she is "in charge" or — more specifically — single-handedly responsible for determining when the couple has sex. Remember: Neither one of you is fertile on your own. At a minimum, I therefore coach my couples on how to ensure that the husband explicitly reassures his wife that he understands she is not "in control" of her cycle. If they experience a frustrating or confusing chart, it is very important that the husband take the lead in making sure the wife does not somehow blame herself for the biological data reflected on the chart. Because while it is the case that the woman is shaped in many ways by the fluctuations and surges of hormones in her body, at the end of the day couples need to admit that this is a facet of life we cannot manipulate to our own ends.

This gets especially tricky when navigating the ups and downs of a specific cycle chart, which might be fairly predictable or may be surprising and frustrating. Unfortunately, there is no single strategy that can guarantee couples will feel comfortable with NFP either short-term or long-term, because NFP is inherently something that is uncomfortable. In a perfect world, where we never fell from perfect grace in the Garden of Eden, there would be no serious need to postpone pregnancy. There would be no illness, no hardship on the woman's body, no financial restrictions, no lack of community support, and no mitigating circumstances that could possibly contribute to anything but a radical welcoming of human life in all its dignity and glory. But that is not the world we live in. And so in order to preserve certain goods like health, finances, and the children we already have, we choose to abstain from another good; namely, sexual intercourse with our spouse. That is not an easy choice, and so there are no easy solutions. But there are particular ways in which we can train ourselves to respond to those difficulties, specifically by drawing on our knowledge of the menstrual cycle as an active force in our marriage. So let me walk through some examples of how couples could step beyond looking at mere biomarkers and include elements of body literacy in your charting experience.

Menstrual phase: Depending on your NFP method, bleeding days may or may not be available for intercourse if you are trying to avoid pregnancy. For women who have particularly difficult periods (e.g., heavy or painful), you may not even desire physical intimacy during this time. However, as the hormones begin to subside and reset, this is a wonderful opportunity to have conversations about family planning intentions. The clarity of mind that accompanies the start of a new cycle is the perfect chance to recommit and reconnect on your values and intentions for this upcoming cycle.

Follicular phase: This is typically a great time for higher-energy dates to spark and rekindle connection between spouses. Regardless of family planning intention, making time to nurture shared hobbies and interests during this phase can ensure that your relationship remains well-rounded and strong. This doesn't have to mean you plan large, elaborate date nights out, but leaning into each other's love languages during this time will avoid the pitfalls of treating sex as a "chore" if you are trying to conceive, or straining the relationship too thin if you are trying to postpone pregnancy.

Ovulatory phase: This is the worst possible time to think in a clearheaded way about family planning intentions. A woman's libido is typically highest during these few days, and her body is producing pheromones that will also make her even more attractive to her spouse. I find that couples who have said they need to postpone pregnancy will sometimes spontaneously choose to switch intentions mid-cycle — which, in and of itself, is not a concern! Of course the Holy Spirit can speak through hormones, and we can never suggest that couples are not free to plan their families however they discern! This can become problematic, however, in the event that either spouse feels anxiety, regret, or even shame in the days following a "change in plans," which then contributes to discord. I tend to suggest to couples that, in the event they feel called to change course mid-cycle, they might want to consider acknowledging that prompting and praying about it together, without acting on it in the moment. If the desire remains at the start of the next cycle, then they can be confident about their discernment going forward.

Luteal phase: This is typically the phase in which couples will experience the most variation in their communication. As women approach their periods, they may feel more physical discomfort, and they may also experience more heightened emotional responses. Both of these things can make it challenging to navigate all aspects of a married relationship, including sexual intimacy. Due to a number of factors, spontaneous sexual desire may be decreased during this phase, which means that husbands and wives must work to cultivate a communal environment in which responsive sexual desire is nurtured instead. This means working with each other to make sure that external stressors (work, a messy house, lingering to-do items) are taken care of so you have the mental and emotional space to relax.

LIVING CYCLICALLY AS HUSBAND AND WIFE
Over the years, my husband and I have worked out some pretty great systems to make sure that we each get some period of reliable sleep. When we had newborns, we split night shifts to make sure that the other person would be able to sleep for at least four hours at a time. Since I'm the night owl, I always took the 10:30 p.m.–2:30 a.m. shift, and my husband took the 2:30–6:30 a.m. shift. As the kids got older and slept better, we instituted a weekend sleep-in schedule. He would get up with the kids on Saturday morning while I slept in, and I would reciprocate by letting him sleep in on Sundays. We still do this, many years later, and it's a nice little routine we have carved out to help make sure that we're both taking care of our health in this small way.

But imagine my surprise one Sunday morning to discover that I was still in bed when my husband had already gotten up and taken care of all of the kids' breakfast needs! I stumbled down the stairs, apologetic and a bit confused. "I'm so sorry, I should have been the one to get up early. I don't know what happened. Is everything okay?"

My husband smiled and simply said, "Everything is fine. I just know that it's day two of your cycle, and that's a day when you're usually really tired. So I thought I'd let you sleep in."

I typically tell this story during my Cycle Prep live programs, to illustrate what it means for us to create a "Culture of Care" for one another. You can probably imagine the looks on the faces of all the moms in attendance, who are sensing, just as I did in that moment, what an incredible gift that was for my husband to give! Not only did he let me sleep in for a little longer, but he took initiative to help me care for my body at a time when my energy levels were really low and I definitely needed the rest. To top it off, this conversation happened in the presence of our children — some of whom were old enough to understand what "day two of your cycle" meant. So he also gave our children the incredible gift of modeling respect for the needs of others. If we take seriously the notion that the two become "one flesh" through marriage (see Gn 2:24), then a husband and wife will experience cyclicality in their union, as their communication styles and interactions shift with the ebb and flow of a woman's cycle. In this way, we can see how family life is an incarnation, so to speak, of the spiritual reality that men become "cyclical creatures" through the grace of the sacraments.

This is something that couples can easily observe even without cycle charting, because there are some times when arguments or tempers tend to flare more easily, just as there are times when communication and cooperation tend to come more naturally. Our previous discussion about virtue applies here, because we must always be mindful to cultivate positive communication in our relationship, regardless of whatever "flavor" of our personality may be asserting itself. But as I said in a recent talk to a young adult group — cycle awareness allows us to understand why sometimes disagreements are more likely to end in shouting, and why other times they are more likely to end in tears!

I wanted to make sure that I heard some men's voices on this topic, so I interviewed men and asked them what they thought the impact of cycle charting has been on their marriage, besides simply knowing about their fertile window for conception. Here are a few responses that really stood out to me:

"NFP has allowed me to understand my wife's cycle and her emotions. Since the day we learned about NFP over eight years ago … our communication has improved significantly. NFP has allowed me to have more empathy, especially when she goes through situations that impact her life and ultimately her cycle."

"I think [cycle charting] has helped me to understand her emotional state and how it changes throughout the month. Knowing a little about her cycle has helped me to be more intentional about loving her."

"In feeling my own emotions, I feel that I am able to tell when she is close to [ovulation] based on how much I want to have sex. For instance, if she [ovulates around] day fifteen, that is when my sexual desire is highest. And during her peak it even is more than say, day nineteen or twenty, when it has been longer since we had sex. Knowing this about myself can help me also redirect my energy to love my wife in other ways."

"Perhaps this is more perspective, but [cycle charting] has given me the logic by which to afford space or attentive care. It also just adds to my appreciation for my wife so that these cycles are a gift by which to mark moments for connection rather than moments of confusion and emotional distress."

A common thread through all of these comments is the idea that marriage is better when the husband understands his wife. I would hope this is just basic common sense, but I also know that many men and women have never been invited to take cycles into account to serve their relationship in this way. Is it necessary for marital harmony for women to chart their cycles? By now you can anticipate that my answer is a resounding "no." But at a minimum, we see that men who are attentive to their wives' cyclical patterns feel more confident understanding her and are better equipped to understand themselves in response.

> *Marriage is better when the husband understands his wife.*

As one respondent shared, "My wife has her cycle, and that's part of who she is. It's the mystery of her own body — her own sacredness — and I don't want to chip away from that. I want her to have it as her own, but as a married couple, it's also *ours* now, and we're both invested in it."

For some couples, leaning into cyclical rhythms will entail making adjustments to your shared routines, or making space in routines that are attentive and responsive to the woman's hormonal shifts. At a minimum, living "cyclically" in a family means that bodily care for a woman's cycle needs will be taken into consideration with at least the same amount of gravitas as other times when our body needs extra rest or attention — like when any member of the family is sick or injured, or in need of extra rest and calories when they are going through a growth spurt. You can easily see how cultivating this aspect of a marriage relationship will naturally flow down to relationships with and among children.

I frequently remind parents that our families are the first school of body literacy: They are the first place our children observe and learn about how we should speak and act to show respect for the function and dignity of our bodies. Through the menstrual cycle, women are given regular opportunities to be intentional about asking for care, and the rest of the family is given regular opportunities to respond generously and lovingly to those requests. Wives: This means you need to be willing to ask for help, and not too proud to graciously receive that help from others. Husbands: This means taking her requests seriously and being willing to adapt when the situation calls for change.

ALLOWING OURSELVES TO BE SEEN

In our previous chapter about Mary, we touched on this idea of "hiddenness" as an aspect of drawing closer to God. We spoke of how there is a meaningful distinction between hiding *from* and hiding *with* God — the former being the posture of Adam and Eve in their shame, and the latter being the posture of the Blessed Virgin Mary. As we conclude this section about cycles and marriage, it's fitting for us to simply meditate on how embracing our cycles as "one flesh" can help us regain some aspect of what was lost between Adam and Eve at the time of the Fall.

Some women are naturally very comfortable and open about sharing their cycle information with their spouse. Others are not. Likewise, some men are very comfortable and open about receiving this information, whereas others are not. Most of this is likely a matter of conditioning: Our reactions and thoughts about these topics typically reflect what we grew up with, and what our experiences have been with cycles and periods up to the point of marriage. Unfortunately, this means that some couples will have a harder time breaking down certain barriers in order to cultivate a shared experience of cyclical living. This is perhaps the strongest case I can make for early cycle education for both young men and young women — because inviting young people to consider this element of women's biology through a positive, faith-directed lens can help make the transition to shared charting much easier. But regardless of whatever path a couple takes to learn about cycles, it is my hope and sincere prayer that they will encounter their cyclical, shared fertility — this hidden element of their marriage that only they intimately know — as an opportunity to draw closer to God.

This is not an easy thing to accomplish, because our society has not necessarily equipped men or women to see cycles with positivity. Understandably, women can sometimes be afraid to share this aspect of their femininity with their husbands, because we have either internalized negative things about ourselves or are worried that negativity will be reflected back to us through our husbands. Regardless of whether our thoughts are positive or negative about our cycles, it is a very vulnerable and intimate thing to share them with someone else.

> *Regardless of whether our thoughts are positive or negative about our cycles, it is a very vulnerable and intimate thing to share them with someone else.*

In closing, I would therefore like to add another set of reflections from husbands who were asked what they would say to a woman who may think negatively about her cycles. Let these words be a positive example of how our Church can help marriages more fully reflect the image of Christ and his Bride, through growing in understanding and appreciation of menstrual cycles:

"I think many of us have parts of who we are that we wish were different. I don't mean to downplay the unique nature of a women's menstrual cycle by saying that. While I have some understanding of it through my wife, I haven't and never will experience it. I mean to say — I know it is hard, but try to be kind to yourself because it is part of who you are and part of the beautiful mystery of being a woman — even if dealing with it and experiencing it doesn't make it feel beautiful or good at all."

"It is so important for [women] to know that [they are] wonderfully made, created by God to be the place of new creation, a

sacred design from the mind of God, not a product of chance and time, random mutation and natural selection."

"As a man, I have NO IDEA how these changes affect anyone other than my wife. I guess I would have to acknowledge that it must be difficult and that I am sorry this is a struggle. In the case where someone is thinking negatively about herself, though, I would remind her that our worth is not in what we do or cannot do, but that we are good because God made us that way. Whenever someone, including myself, thinks negatively about themselves, I try to remind people of that fact. There is nothing we can do, or that happens to us, that makes us bad. God made us good; we need to claim it!"

"Cycles can be healthy for any relationship. I think of our relationship with God, which has time for feasts around Christmas and Easter and times for fasting with Lent and Advent. In the same way the relationship between a couple when in the fertile or non-fertile periods can help create a cycle. There can be times of desire and absence, and there can be times of feasting. Sometimes they are bittersweet; other times they help create desire and love in the relationship."

CHAPTER 15

Transitions

As we begin to wrap up our thoughts on the *language of the body* through menstrual cycles, let's return to a concept that we discussed earlier in the book — namely, the reality that women go through three different stages, or phases, in their reproductive lives. We previously discussed a sort of parallel between the reproductive life of a woman and the "reproductive" life of the Church through her sacraments. The crucifixion of Jesus Christ can be likened to a girl's first shedding of blood at menarche, while menopause is mirrored in the end of the Church's reproductive life at the coming of the New Jerusalem and the fulfillment of the kingdom of God. Let's return to these ideas, so that we can reflect now on those particular times of transition in our female bodies. Is there a way that embracing and understanding the entrance and exit of our cycles can also lead us deeper into self-knowledge and, consequently, love of God? As the *language of the body* shifts through these different stages, how do we help girls and women positively integrate these bodily experiences (as uncomfortable and confusing as they may be!) into their experience of God's unique and unrepeatable love for them?

I take for granted that most of my readers will have already experienced puberty and gone through this first time of transition, but I'm guessing that many will not yet have gone through perimenopause and are therefore anticipating this second transition still. What I would therefore like to do is first invite us to think about how what we have learned and explored in this book can help us navigate this second transition into menopause. How can we think positively about the way the *language of our body* shifts during this time? What do we need from the Church in order to better understand this aspect of our femininity? What practical support might we need to navigate these changes? And then we'll wrap up with an exploration of how we, as Church, can provide better accompaniment to the next generation of girls as they enter the first transition into cyclical life at puberty.

Before offering some deeper reflection, let us begin by looking at what is happening at the biological level during these times of transition. How are they similar, but also how are they different?

Menarche and Menopause

The onset of a girl's first vaginal bleed is called *menarche*. I chose not to say "a girl's first period" because it's entirely possible that a girl's first experience of a bleed is not actually a true period — meaning that it was not preceded by ovulation, but is instead reflecting other hormonal activity as her body is trying to learn how to produce its first ovulation. This is not the level of granular detail that I discuss with nine-year-olds in my programming, but it's an important point to make here because it speaks to the fact that the process of beginning our menstrual cycles is a sort of liminal, or in-between, state. During puberty, a girl's body needs to learn how to coordinate all of the different hormone cascades and activities that together make up a full menstrual cycle.

A girl's first bleed is therefore not the end of the puberty process, but rather an indication that her body has begun the complicated process of maturing its hypothalamic-pituitary-ovarian axis, which is sort of like the control system for regulating menstrual cycles. This HPO axis is a complicated channel of communication between various hormone-producing and -regulating aspects of our body, all of which work together to synchronize and create a menstrual cycle. In my teen charting program, I liken it to a basketball team, which is made up of individual players who all need to learn how to work together. For that to happen, they simply need time to practice. Teens' cycles are therefore irregular in the first few years because the various "team members" haven't quite perfected the ways they work together yet. But they're figuring it out, and that's okay.

Another way to think about it is like a carousel: When we first get on a carousel, the ride begins very slowly and gradually works up to speed. This is similar to what happens when a girl begins her menstrual cycles — the first few years should be seen as the first few revolutions on a carousel, which are slower but gradually getting faster as it gets up to speed.

Because of their transitional nature, teen cycles inherently come with more variations and some more complications than more mature cycles. The upper bound for "normal" women's cycle lengths is typically stated to be around thirty-five days; however, it's not uncommon for teens to go as long as forty-five days in a single cycle and sometimes as long as sixty days. Teens also have more frequent anovulatory bleeds than grown women and are more susceptible to heavy periods, painful periods, and — thanks to a combination of growth spurts and frequent, heavy bleeds — anemia. Puberty certainly cannot be distilled down to the processes directly related to our menstrual cycle, but if we think about it sort of like "peri-menarche" — or the years around menarche — then it becomes more clear that we should expect these cycle irregularities as a normal way our growing bodies learn to figure all of this out.

In thinking this way, we can more easily see the parallel between the first transitional time of puberty and what is sometimes called "second puberty" later in life. Women officially enter menopause when we have not had a period bleed for at least one year. Before that time, most women will experience many years of what we call *perimenopause* — the time surrounding menopause. These years actually mirror the first few years of puberty, which we spoke of being like the experience of a carousel "winding up." As our cycles "wind down," it therefore makes sense that we'll start to see a lot of irregularity and other changes popping up with our cycles. The process isn't exactly parallel, but varying cycle lengths and changes in bleeding patterns that previously reflected an HPO axis that was trying to establish communication are now going to reflect an HPO axis in which communication is sort of breaking down.

Just like puberty, this process tends to take a few years. And like puberty, women need to remember that everyone's timeline is going to be unique — while most women enter perimenopause in their early forties, some women don't begin the process in earnest until closer to the age of fifty, and some women can start seeing signs as early as age thirty-five and would still not be considered premature in their transition. To complicate things even further, menopause can also be brought about surgically or sometimes chemically through the loss of ovarian function during chemotherapy — in which case there is very little transition time at all. How can the Church do a better job of accompanying girls and women through the vast array of experiences that go with these transitions?

The Perimenopause Transition — Moving Beyond Cycles
In my line of work as an NFP instructor, I have spoken with so many women who worry about what perimenopause will bring. They are anxious about hot flashes, mood swings, the unpredictability of their cycles, and many other normal body changes that can, admittedly, make perimenopause a challenging time. Yet there is also an element of expectation and hope, because cycles and periods are certainly not easy all the time. When I have surveyed women prior to my perimenopause presentations, about sixty percent of them admit that they have a mix of both positive and negative emotions when they think about menopause. Even though many of them are somewhat eager for cycles to stop, there is also a sense that without those cycles, a familiar element of their life will be lost. Through menopause, women are aware that we will experience a sort of "dying" of our reproductive self — something our male counterparts do not go through to the same degree. This can be a particularly difficult challenge for women who have struggled with infertility or for women who have not gotten married (even those who have chosen not to do so), because it also begs a final acceptance of life on earth without the fruits of biological children.

This is one area where the transition of perimenopause is very different from puberty: In our early teens, the majority of our years are likely still ahead of us. Vocational paths have not yet been discerned, and most pubertal girls have very little life experience to draw on. Our brains haven't even matured enough to synthesize our bodily experiences with deeper questions on the meaning of our existence. But in perimenopause, we are grown women who collectively inhabit very different vocational spheres! Some of us have been married for decades and others are single, either because of a choice to join consecrated single life or because we are still waiting in hope for that state-of-life vocation to be made clear. Children may not be in the picture at all, or there may already be grandchildren to account for. And obviously there can be all sorts of gradations in between. Coupled with a growing awareness of our own mortality, the sort of person who enters perimenopause is, quite simply, a much more complicated individual than the girl who entered puberty. What is the truth that we need to hear about our femininity during this time of transition? What do perimenopausal women need from the Church?

The first area the Church can be of assistance is in the practical realm of education. Shifts in our cycles will likely mean that married women who are using Natural Family Planning will need support in order to navigate this transition with their husbands. This applies to couples who may be trying to postpone pregnancy in these final years of fertility, but also to couples who are actively trying to conceive during this time. Even if couples have been confidently charting together for decades, this is typically a moment when they might need to reconnect with a previous instructor or consider switching to a new method altogether. So it is important for our Church — and here I am specifically thinking about local parishes — to provide information about NFP resources and related couples' ministries to the community at large, rather than myopically focusing on family planning as a topic of interest to engaged couples. The Church's willingness to serve as a place where education is offered and generously provided can go a very long way toward serving women in this important time.

For women who are unmarried (even religious sisters!), access to programs to teach cycle charting can also be hugely important, because the age at which we go through perimenopause also corresponds to a time in life when other health concerns may begin to pop up. Certain cancers, thyroid issues, insulin resistance leading to diabetes, and many other things can manifest during this time — and they can also lead to certain cycle changes. We shouldn't just assume that every change we experience during perimenopause is directly related to that transition. We need ways to articulate and communicate with doctors about the constellation of symptoms we are experiencing, so they can help us understand and investigate whether there are other issues going on besides the breakdown of menstrual cycles. And let's be honest: It's incredibly unlikely with our current healthcare system that a doctor's office is going to provide the education and support needed to do this. So this is one area where the Church can truly lean into her dual mission of educating the mind and caring for the body, by ensuring that valuable information about cycle health is offered to all women, not just those in certain vocational situations.

Additionally, the Church needs to be a space where the goodness and beauty of womanhood is proclaimed through perimenopause and beyond. Society is typically very negative about this time of transition, so it's very easy for women to absorb negative or shameful views about ourselves if we don't have a voice reminding us who we actually are, in the eyes of God. Women can particularly struggle with sexuality at this time of life, both because of our culture's distorted views on the topic and because what we primarily hear in the Church about sex has to do with fertility. So to counter the latter issue, the Church as a whole can be better about articulating that sexual intercourse between spouses is still good, beautiful, and fruitful beyond the time of reproductive age. I have heard from more than a few couples that it was difficult to switch their mentality about sex after menopause, because it meant that there was no longer a balance between the unitive and procreative aspects to consider. While it's admittedly somewhat fun and freeing, overly scrupulous couples have worried that sex without the possibility of more children is somehow wrong, so we need to be aware of that dynamic when ministering to couples in this stage of life. While intentional sterilization is never condoned by the Church, the natural sterility that comes about through menopause is never an impediment to spousal unity.

Yet our acceptance of God's natural design should also include the gentle acceptance that sexual function for both partners can decline with age, and there is nothing wrong with either partner if their bodies' sexual response does not function the same way it did when they were younger. This is where the voice of society must be tempered, because far too often women are encouraged to reject the process of aging and attempt to override our bodies' design in order to achieve a glamorized notion that menopause should be a time of "sexual liberation" for us. Even before that time, doctors often suggest sterilization in order to navigate perimenopause without the "threat" of unplanned pregnancy. Or couples who are trying to conceive will be counseled on fertility treatments that do not honor the natural design of our bodies. So our Church needs to counter these cultural lies that put undue importance on recreational sex and prey on the fears and desires of couples who are navigating this transition in their shared fertility.

In articulating a balance between both of these aspects of marital intimacy post-menopause, our faith can thus pave the way for women to better see that our worth as "wife" is not tied to our biological ability to conceive and bear children. This same message is also needed for women going through perimenopause who are unmarried, because it is a reminder that the dignity of woman can and should be understood independent of her reproductive potential with a man. We discussed earlier in the book that the complementarity of man and woman is one part of how we image God, but that this complementarity must be preceded by an understanding of the individual way we *image* God in our womanhood. Another way of saying this is that our identity as *daughter of God* is of more importance than our identity as *wife of man.* So let's meditate on that identity as it is uniquely experienced in this transitional time of perimenopause.

DAUGHTERS OF GOD

After having experienced the ups and downs of cycle phases for so many years, along with the constantly shifting energy and mood levels, post-menopausal women will often say that they experience a sort of liberation, or even a second childhood. Lara Briden articulates this in her book *The Hormone Repair Manual*, as she reflects on research by Harvard psychologist Emily Hancock: "Girls crystalize their most authentic sense of self sometime between the ages of 8 and 10. After that, Hancock says, puberty arrives, and girls can often start to feel the pressure of the female gender role. ... The process can reverse at menopause when women have an opportunity to reconnect with the inner girl."[1]

When I read this, I was struck particularly by this idea that women who have entered menopause could become more "child-like." For Christians, it is hard to hear that phrase and not imagine Jesus' words: "Truly, I say to you, whoever does not receive the kingdom of God like a child shall not enter it" (Mk 10:15).

Of course, Jesus does not mean that only children can enter heaven. He does not mean that we must literally age backward and become children again in order to enter the kingdom of God. Like Nicodemus, who struggled to understand Jesus' teaching on spiritual rebirth, we may find ourselves scratching our heads and wondering: "How can a man be born when he is old? Can he enter a second time into his mother's womb and be born?" (Jn 3:4). How could it be that, for women, the physical act of aging and losing our cycles is something that can help restore elements of our youth?

Whenever there appears to be a paradox such as this, it is important for Catholics to lean in and seek the wisdom of God to help us understand. We have already spoken of the symbolism that we can find through menopause as it relates to the life of the Church. Post-menopausal women reflect the idea that our Church will also cease her liturgical cycles when the Bride has reached her full maturity in the New Jerusalem. But is there a way in which this biological event can also inform and deepen our sense of self, and our relationship with God?

I imagine that, as with everything we have discussed so far, each woman will have a unique experience with God and self as her cycles lengthen and eventually disappear. But I'd like to offer two key ideas worthy of reflection as we ponder what it could mean for mature women to become more childlike.

First, we can think about the energy, creativity, and zeal of childhood. Contrary to the perimenopausal propensity for feeling tired and worn out, many women emerge into menopause with a sense of invigoration and energy. Briden points out that "the Japanese word for menopause is *kounenki,* which translates as 'renewal years' or 'energy.'"[2]

It is often the case that post-menopausal women will want to pick up a new hobby, or suddenly encounter a newfound delight in activities that did not interest them before — a trait that does strike this mother of young children as being particularly childlike. Chesterton writes about the energy and vitality of children as one specific way that they image God. To him, God is childlike in the sense that he never grows weary of repetition, or of taking delight in the little things. "It may be that He has the eternal appetite of infancy," Chesterton writes, "for we have sinned and grown old, and our Father is younger than we."[3] Perhaps the neurological changes that accompany menopause are a way in which grown women are invited to regain this sort of childlike wonder, which may have been hidden or suppressed by the hormonal shifts of menstrual cycles.

Of course, we must also be prudent and not adopt the attitude that puberty and our subsequent reproductive years somehow inhibit women from experiencing and living out a true version of ourselves. Countless female saints have shown us that authentic holiness — which is, simply put, the full flourishing of the human person — can be achieved at any age and in any circumstance. We must be clear on that, even as we articulate a positive vision for how Christian women can draw closer to God in and through menopause.

Second, we can revisit Matthew's telling of the story of Jesus welcoming the little children, in which Jesus specifically explains to the crowd that to be childlike is to be "humble" (Mt 18:4). Humility is not about self-deprecation, but rather being able to see oneself clearly — to admit that even though we are small and insignificant compared with God, we are inestimably loved and cared for by our Creator.

Perimenopause is certainly a time when women come face to face with the fact that we are simply not in control of all that happens with our bodies — and all of these physical changes and challenges are compounded because they coincide with a number of other significant life changes. Careers may be shifting, children may be leaving the house, and new caretaker roles tend to emerge — for our own aging parents, for a new generation of grandchildren, or sometimes both!

To be humble during this time is to put our full trust in God to provide, for we know our own littleness and can perceive our need for his loving care. As the preacher Simon Tugwell wrote, "The Lord is not suggesting that heaven is a great playground for Arcadian infants. The children are our model because they have no claim on heaven. If they are close to God, it is because they are incompetent … there is no question of their having yet been able to merit anything. If they receive anything, it can only be as a gift."[4]

When we think about humility in this way, we can see how the time of perimenopause and menopause are natural moments when God invites us to perceive our own littleness, but also to ponder and trust in his great care for us. Of course, this can be said of any major life event, and in this respect perimenopause is not unique; but we are invited to experience this time of change as a time of being held, comforted, and nurtured by our loving Father.

This can be an especially poignant thing to reflect upon during this time of transition, because this is also the first time that some women are going through a new phase in life without their mother's guidance. For women who have lost their mothers, the transition of perimenopause reveals new facets of grief — which is something that, as an NFP instructor, I was initially surprised by because I had not considered it. When we think about times when girls need their mothers, what usually comes to mind are times like puberty, pregnancy, and early motherhood. We don't usually consider perimenopause as one such time, but a connection back to our own childhood can be opened up in a powerful way as we go through this experience.

Here we also see an invitation for the Church to truly fulfill that role of "mother" — not in any formal way through liturgy or rites, but through her unique understanding of and ability to care for the human person. At the most basic level, Catholic women desire and deserve community in which to explore the biological changes that are happening alongside other shifts in body image, relationships, and even our prayer lives! It is unlikely, perhaps, to think that women would want to form a sort of Bible study or prayer group specifically focused on perimenopause. That would probably make most of us feel reduced to our reproductive status. But at a minimum, we should not shy away from this topic! As we have discussed, the biological dimension of cycles cannot be siphoned off of our concept of "womanhood." In order to approach God with our whole selves, we need to be affirmed and encouraged to do so with not just our souls, heart, and minds, but our bodies as well.

THE MENARCHE TRANSITION

Having thought a little more about what we might desire from the Church as we navigate the transition of perimenopause, let's talk about what we might want to provide in our support for girls as they go through the first transition of puberty. Unlike adult women who have the maturity and life experience to question not just the practical aspects but also the deeper *meaning* of cycle changes, girls going through puberty often need guidance in smaller, more practical steps. Intuitively, it doesn't make sense to ask a nine-year-old girl with breast buds to contemplate her body's symbolic signification of God as a nursing mother (see Is 49). But as most of us reflect on our own puberty experience and think about what would have served us better in our adult lives, an overwhelming majority of women come to the conclusion that the education could simply have been better.

So now let us ask ourselves: If the Church is going to pave the way for young women to truly embrace their femininity in and through their bodily functions, what do we want those girls to know? How do we want their experience to be different from ours? What parts of puberty could have been more positive?

In perimenopause, it seems there is no societal standard for education: Women are largely left to research the process ourselves or talk with our doctors individually. But for puberty, there are built-in opportunities to educate girls so they don't have to figure things out on their own. Schools will typically offer at least some basic education on pubertal development; however, there is admittedly a lot that is lacking — and much that is completely misguided — in many of these approaches. In many cases, proximate education on puberty happens in fourth or fifth grade and includes an "everything all at once" approach. Boys and girls are separated (although in many cases this is no longer the norm!) and all the girls are taught about breast buds, bras, hair growth, body odor, periods, sexual reproduction, STI's and pregnancy prevention in one single sitting. I received this sort of presentation in school and remember fairly little of it, but I do know that what I learned about periods did not prepare me at all for the experience I had at menarche. I didn't understand how my body actually works and what goes on to produce a period bleed. I didn't know what was normal for a teen to experience and when I should be talking to a doctor.

If I had received less support from home, or had already felt uncomfortable in my changing body, I could see how that sort of experience would be disorienting and would be something that a girl would want to suppress or alter. To put it bluntly: I believe that poor education and support could actually lead to a dissociating experience with one's body during puberty. And we have research that shows that education which adequately prepares girls for the start of menarche can lead to a decrease in anxiety and an overall better experience with puberty.[5] So if we are serious about helping our girls (and boys!) navigate this transition positively, we cannot neglect the very concrete call to provide quality education.

But what is the role of the Church in this? Let's start with the family, which — mirroring the Church's language — I like to call the first school of body literacy. What should parents know about shepherding their daughters through this transition of menarche?

WHAT GIRLS AND PARENTS SHOULD KNOW ABOUT MENARCHE

We have already discussed in our introductory chapters how cycles are considered to be a fifth vital sign for girls, meaning they are an important part of assessing a girl's overall health. So, for a family to be adequately equipped to navigate cycles, they would need to understand a few things, some of which we have already covered in this book. Specifically, families should help their daughters learn:

The science of the menstrual cycle
Going through some of the details in chapter 1 of this book could be great.

Options for period products and management
Most moms are most comfortable having their girls start with pads, but new options like period underwear and even period swimwear could be great additions. Parents and girls will also have different comfort levels with insertable devices like tampons, cups, or discs. I always suggest in my workshops that girls should defer to the guidance and wisdom of their mothers if there are strong preferences, but parents also should be aware that using an insertable device does not "violate" a girl's innocence at all. Virginity cannot be lost through insertion of a menstrual product.

Normal and abnormal variations for teens
Let your daughter know that irregularity is normal at first! Teach her that symptoms such as pain or severe mood swings are not things she needs to hide or deal with on her own, and that you are willing to help her get relief. You can also teach her about cervical fluid as a healthy sign, so she can quickly learn to identify any signs of change that might indicate a vaginal infection, specifically.

Common cycle issues that manifest in the teen years
Teens do typically experience heavier and more painful periods due to the immaturity of their HPO axis and the balance of

hormones in adolescence, but issues such as endometriosis and PCOS can also manifest during this time. In speaking with pediatricians, I've been told that teens are also especially prone to amenorrhea (the loss of periods) due to rigorous sports schedules, and even anemia due to the confluence of growth spurts and heavy bleeds.

Options for tracking cycles to identify abnormalities or areas of potential concern
Whether she tracks cycles with a notebook, calendar, paper chart, or app, a girl should understand that "period tracking" is really just tracking bleeds and can't give a lot of meaningful information about whether she is ovulating or her cycle phases are showing signs of overall balance. I don't think that all girls need to chart their cycles, but being invited to do so allows her to begin gaining valuable knowledge about her body right from the start.

Having this foundation in biology is a crucial step toward future conversations that will help our children understand and appreciate the inherent dignity, health, and goodness of their sexual body functions. Without understanding how our bodies work and what they were designed to do, it's very hard to explain the Catholic view of chastity and the meaning of sexual intimacy within marriage. Additionally, an appreciation for the natural vocation to marriage effectively paves the way for vocations that do not include sexual reproduction: namely, consecrated life and the priesthood. We have already posited that our theological understanding of spiritual fatherhood and motherhood will be enriched if we are able to interpret the "sexual" meaning of our bodies in light of the dimension of sign, apart from being limited to their reproductive function. Religious brothers, sisters, and fathers are not exempt from the need to understand and appreciate their embodied goodness. On the contrary, I believe our

Church should especially insist that formation and education in consecrated or priestly life should predispose the individual to joyfully accept their physical nature as integral to their unique image of God. According to the *Catechism*, "In the consecrated life, Christ's faithful, moved by the Holy Spirit, propose to follow Christ more nearly, to give themselves to God who is loved above all and, pursuing the perfection of charity in the service of the Kingdom, to signify and proclaim in the Church the glory of the world to come."[6] We must prepare our brothers and sisters to give themselves completely in whatever state of life God calls them — a task that must include the physical elements of self, including the transition of puberty.

Honestly, I think all families should have the opportunity to receive and hand on this practical information for their daughters. But specifically for Catholic families, this information needs to be presented in a way that either directly and explicitly ties it to our Faith, or at least utilizes a Christian approach to body positivity: reverence for the goodness and dignity of the body with respect for natural biological function.

BODY POSITIVE EDUCATION

The term "body positivity" started popping up in the late 1990s and since then has grown into a larger movement, specifically in terms of advertising and media. At its core, the body positivity movement is about recognizing the good aspects of various body shapes and types, rather than exclusively forwarding one "ideal" image. The primary goal is to help people focus less on comparing their outward appearances to arbitrary — and sometimes harmful — cultural norms, and more on health, both physical and emotional. On the surface, this project harmonizes beautifully with the Christian understanding of respect for the body. In particular, Catholics can benefit from paying close attention to research that indicates that our educational programming should address the *emotional* aspects of preparation in order to improve our girls' attitudes toward and experience of menarche.[7] We need only take the movement one step further to include spiritual health, so our girls can begin the important process of integrating all of these aspects.

True body positivity must always be tempered so that it never loses sight of this integral vision of health. There have been worries recently that body positivity includes an "everything goes" approach to praising our bodies, even to the point of neglecting the goal of integrated health. So how can Christian parents, specifically, pass along what is good about these body positivity movements, without leading our children to a sort of quasi-body worship? Christian author Jess Connolly puts forward the following idea:

> We can speak positive words towards our bodies while also acknowledging they're broken, that they're subject to the effect of a world that is not God's best-case scenario. What's more, it's not our bodies that we worship or proclaim as perfect as much as it is the God who made our bodies … The statement that I love my body, that I feel positively about it, has so much more *impact* because it's backed up by the belief that the Creator of the universe made it with intention and creativity.[8]

Connolly's insights are articulated from the standpoint of someone who has been able to guide, inform, and integrate her body image through the lens of faith. From my experience, this is something that many teenagers are not quite ready to do in a mature way yet, but that doesn't mean we can't lay the foundation for them to be able to articulate these things later in life. So how can we use body positive language, infused with the values of our faith, to help insulate our children from negative self-image, especially in these sensitive teen years?

When I speak with parents, I give examples of very easy ways we can shape our language about menstruation — and bodily function in general — to help our children have a more positive attitude about their bodies during the puberty transition. I suggest using words that equate goodness with healthy function, rather than physical appearance. It's also important to emphasize that each person's body is "smart." Our bodies know what a healthy developmental timeline looks like for us, and have ways of communicating to us about whether something is not quite right — we just need to respect our bodies enough to listen!

Here are some sample sentences I offer to illustrate this point:

- A menstrual cycle is important, hard work that girls' and women's bodies do!
- Periods are a visible sign that your body is doing exactly what it was designed to do.
- Menstrual cycles are important to girls' and women's health.
- Pain is a sign that your body is communicating something. Be sure to pay attention to the signals your body gives you!
- Period blood is good, healthy blood.
- Don't worry about comparing yourself to your friends. Your body knows the right timeline for you to be on for puberty. Your body knows what is healthy for you.

I encourage parents to avoid the common phrases "late bloomer" or "early bloomer" when I am talking about puberty. Inherent in these words is the idea that puberty is about transforming from a bud into a flower. And while the analogy can somewhat be supported, the message girls receive when hearing this is that going through puberty makes you attractive. It makes you more beautiful. It makes you an object worthy to behold. But to her loving Father, is a girl any less attractive, beautiful, or worthy of beholding than a full-grown woman? Of course not.

Thus, when we educate our girls about their periods, we should be attentive not only to the content we are providing, but also to the way in which that content is delivered. These suggestions apply equally to fathers as they do to mothers. While many of the direct conversations about puberty and periods do happen between mothers and daughters, we know that this is not always the case! Some dads are in the unique position of needing to be the one who explains these aspects of puberty to their daughters. Some parents always try to have puberty conversations with their kids together. I'm sure there are also some families in which Dad is more comfortable talking about these things. But regardless of who says what and how the direct conversations happen, it's important for both parents to lead the way modeling positive language around our children's changing bodies and responding generously when she does approach for help.

PRIMARY EDUCATORS AND THEIR SUPPORT SYSTEMS

The Church has consistently declared and repeated that parents are the primary educators of their children, especially in matters of virtue, morality, and faith. One of the clearest documents to express this is the 1995 guide "The Truth and Meaning of Human Sexuality," written by the Pontifical Council for the Family. It states, "The role of parents in education is of such importance that it is almost impossible to find an adequate substitute. It is therefore the duty of parents to create a family atmosphere inspired by love and devotion to God and their fellow-men which will promote an integrated, personal and social education of their children."[9] The document goes on to explain, however, that when the Church speaks of parents as the primary educators, she envisions them as the first voices in a chain of educational subsidiarity:

> This implies the legitimacy and indeed the need of giving assistance to the parents, but finds its intrinsic and absolute limit in their prevailing right and their actual capabilities. The principle of subsidiarity is thus at the service of parental love, meeting the good of the family unit. For parents by themselves are not capable of satisfying every requirement of the whole process of raising children, especially in matters concerning their schooling and the entire gamut of socialization. Subsidiarity thus complements paternal and maternal love and confirms its fundamental nature, inasmuch as all other participants in the process of education are only able to carry out their responsibilities in the name of the parents, with their consent and, to a certain degree, with their authorization.[10]

Pope St. John Paul II echoes this vision in *Familiaris Consortio* when he says, "The family is the primary but not the only and exclusive educating community" (40). The relationship the Church envisions is one whereby competent educators make themselves available to assist parents in supplementing home education through their unique skills and expertise — not replacing parental guidance, but supporting it. Thus the values of home are reinforced and strengthened through a community of educators, all working together toward the integrated development of the child.

Therefore, I'd like to push back against a notion I often encounter with some Catholic schools and parents, which is a very rigid interpretation of "primary educators" to mean "sole educators." I worry that Catholic institutions either hide behind or are strong-armed into adopting a "parents as primary educators" model for puberty education that neglects the necessity for subsidiary levels of support! Even many Theology of the Body programs for kids and teens do not include modules specifically on puberty, periods, or cycles. Instead of this approach, I believe we — as Church — should be discussing ways in which Catholic institutions can offer education on these topics in conformity with the truth, goodness, and beauty of our bodies' designs — not to override parental voices or insert themselves over and against parents. That would be explicitly contrary to this subsidiarity model. But our institutions should be ensuring that parents who want supporting voices on these topics have a trustworthy place to turn.

In John Paul II's model, subsidiarity exists in order to make sure that the information and values parents are teaching at home are reinforced in other educational spheres; but I also believe that subsidiarity includes the acknowledgment that many parents who firmly intend to provide primary education on these topics do still feel that they need assistance with the finer details. Speaking as a member of the "X-ennial" generation, I can say that the vast majority of my peers received little to no formal education about what actually goes on in a menstrual cycle. If we were lucky, we were told what period flow consisted of, but many of us did not even absorb that much information. And while parents who have been practicing NFP for many years tend to have a fair grasp of the cycles of adult women, they typically have very little knowledge of how teen puberty cycles are different, and what to look for to understand normal and healthy variations in these transitional years. So in these cases, subsidiarity also means that the school, parish, or other educational organization should be providing information that the parent wants to provide, but does not feel equipped to do alone.

I have a very strong preference for shared learning models

of cycle and period education, where programs are delivered simultaneously to parents and children together. In this way, the entire family receives the benefit of skilled teaching and training in these topics, and they also have a shared experience to return to and reference in future conversations. Another way institutions can provide subsidiary support is by giving parents programs to do at home with their child, or they could take a hybrid approach whereby certain elements of a topic are taught at school, and then parents are provided take-home supplements for further learning. Still another way would be parallel learning programs, in which children receive one presentation geared for their age and learning level, while parents receive a presentation that is specifically tailored to them. In short, I see many potential, good solutions to subsidiary education on these topics that all honor the parents' primary role.

So, from the above discussion, we can see that the role of the Church is multifaceted when it comes to helping our girls transition through menarche into adolescence and adult life. It requires the commitment of faithful parents, who take seriously their role as formators and educators in these topics for their children. But it also requires the service of subsidiary levels of education, whereby parents who would like assistance in the more technical aspects of these topics can find suitable aid from sources that they trust.

TRANSEAMUS

Even as we do the important work of crafting practical puberty education models within the Church, I do want to make sure that we maintain a focus on what is truly essential to holiness. The last thing I want is a bunch of parents and school administrators wringing their hands because they feel that they are failing to shepherd our children by not offering the perfect way for boys and girls to understand the *language of the body* in puberty.

We must offer our best efforts, but we will never be perfect, and God is able to work many graces with that. So as we wrap up this section on transitions, I'd like to offer one final reflection.

It can be tempting to think about menarche or menopause as obstacles that we need to overcome in our lives. This is especially true if we focus on how confusing or uncomfortable or frustrating the processes may be. But our Catholic Faith does not see transitions as hurdles to be overcome. Transitions are not bad things we need to get through in order to get back to the path we were supposed to be on. Rather, transitions are bridges that are part of the journey itself, leading us from one good thing to another.

At all times and in all things, God is offering us a particular opportunity for grace. The Latin word "transire" from which we get the word "transition" means a crossing or a passing over, which hopefully holds theological resonances for us because with God, a *passing over* is nothing short of an act of salvation. God says explicitly to the Israelites in Egypt: "When I see the blood, I will pass over you" or, in Latin, *et transibo vos*[11] (Ex 12:13). Christ passed over from life into death, and death back into life — a parallel that was solidified in the early Church through Christ's identity as our Passover lamb. In baptism, we undergo this same crossing over from death into life. In short, transitions carry deep theological significance.

Even more pertinent to our everyday experiences, I'd like to challenge all of us to think about the way in which Christ personally calls us to journey with him through all of the transitions in our lives. Just as we thought about ourselves as daughters of God, being likened to the little children Jesus calls to himself, let us also reflect on our own time of transition echoed in one specific time Jesus asked his disciples to "go across to the other side" (Mk 4:35) with him (in Latin, *transeamus contra*).

Jesus has just spoken at length to the crowds in parables,

speaking to them from beside the sea — but took no time to explain the parables' meanings to them. It is only the disciples, the ones Jesus knows intimately, to whom he explains the meaning and challenges them to deeper understanding. So after departing from the crowd, Jesus invites them all to cross over with him to the other side of the sea, and they all board a boat. While on board, "A great storm of wind arose, and the waves beat into the boat, so that the boat was already filling" (Mk 4:37). They wake Jesus, who calms the storm and thus shows his power.

How many times do we face these transitions, these invitations God gives us to cross over with him, and experience them as real storms in our lives? We may be tempted to think that God has simply fallen asleep at the wheel. We may feel like we've been hoodwinked into getting into a tiny little boat and tossed on the sea, with no clear understanding of why Jesus invited us here in the first place. But it is precisely this crossing over through the peril of the storm that allows us to understand God's power and providence in all things. So let us, like the disciples, heed Christ's invitation to accompany him in these and all of the crossing-overs of our lives — so that he can lead us safely to the other side as we continue the journey with him.

Conclusion

I wish there were a way for an author to see her work in the same way God is able to look upon his work of creation — to know, for certain, that the work is good and to be able to name it as such. One of my favorite lines I've ever read in a writing from the saints comes from Hildegard von Bingen, whom we referenced earlier in this text. At the end of *Cause et cure,* she pens a little pun in Latin on the word *liber* that can mean either "book" or "free": *Explicit iste liber, scriptor sit crimine liber.* "This book ends; may the writer be free from criticism."[1]

Unfortunately, the finitude of human experience means that we will never be able to fully see things the way God does. Instead, the best we can do is to offer up the inevitable imperfections, oversights, and clumsy design of our little creations. I am certain that in the shaping of this particular text, there are innumerable situations that I have not been able to include. We have discussed a mere sliver of the rich tradition our Church has to offer in understanding the nature of the human person as image and likeness of God.

So I hope that my readers will forgive any of those perceived gaps and perhaps craft their own contribution to the work of exploring how science can help us better understand the *language of the body* as a mode of signifying and coming to know God. That's a challenge issued to the Church at large.

But what about you, as a singularly and lovingly crafted daughter of God? After putting down this book, is there a "next step" for you?

Despite barely scratching the surface, this text has covered a lot of ground. Some of the ideas may seem immediately actionable to you, and others may not. Some concepts may resonate with you and provide a natural springboard for contemplation — and others simply may not. Or perhaps they do not resonate with you *yet*.

Body literacy is a skill that takes time to develop and hone, and that process need not be linear. In fact, I would venture to say that growing in body literacy regarding menstrual cycles should decidedly not be thought of as a linear process! It should be thought of as a spiral, in which the same biological and theological realities are revisited numerous times throughout our lives. Each time we revisit a theme, though, the hope is that our understanding will have expanded just a little bit — and we will therefore have drawn just one step closer to our loving Creator.

Having said all of this, I also have a responsibility to make it abundantly clear that no woman is ever required to chart her cycle or even learn about the intricacies of the phases of her menstrual cycle in order to have a deep, beautiful, lasting relationship with God. If I said that, or even slightly intimated that this were the case, I would find myself needing to answer to the countless women saints who have gone before us in faith! In this text, I have put forward some ideas for ways that women can think about how our cycles image God, but I am under no delusions that our cycles are the primary way in which we image God. They are merely *one* facet of embodied femininity, which I have attempted to break open and ponder in light of new, modern knowledge that was previously hidden from our understanding. New knowledge about the designs of creation should always be seen as an opportunity for God's children to take a step back, and attempt to see with God how all that he made is good.

Which brings us back to the question of next steps, and here I feel that it is my duty, having led you so far to the end of this book, to at least provide a little bit of guidance on where you might consider going from here. The suggestions that follow are not sequential steps, but simply a list of options — all of which I think are worthy points for ongoing exploration.

Learn how to chart your cycles

If you have never learned how to chart your unique cycle, here is your invitation to do so. Hopefully this book has given you a good idea of what sort of information you can glean about your cycles by learning to observe biomarkers and track ovulation. The appendix that follows provides some specific information about various methods and resources you could choose, including brief commentary on how to sort through all of these good options in order to find a method that feels comfortable and suits your needs.

Go deeper in your charting practice

So much of this book has been born out of the desire to invite women (and men!) to go beyond a purely pragmatic approach to cycle charting for family planning. I have seen the difference it makes in a marriage and in the practice of NFP when couples see value in charting, rather than simply adopting the practice because the Church tells them they "have to." If you've already been charting your cycles, this could be an opportunity to deepen your practice by just adding one small component to help you grow closer to yourself, God, or even your spouse. For example, if you already know about your cycle patterns, try using that knowledge in a specific way to either improve communication with your spouse, or gain some new insight into your nightly examen. There's no need to go overboard trying to implement everything all at once — just ask yourself where you'd like to grow in body literacy, and see if you can build upon the great foundation you already have.

Incorporate your body into your prayer life
Even if you have no desire to try praying in sync with your cycle phases (which is totally fine, by the way! Have I mentioned that this is totally fine?), you could deepen your understanding of the language of your body simply by being intentional about praying *with* your body. This is encouraged by our Mother Church, not only through her rich sacramental life, which bestows grace through physical actions, but also through the rich tradition of gestures and prayer postures that are woven into the liturgy. These gestures may have shifted over time, but in general we can think about how the Church encourages kneeling, standing, bowing, and making the sign of the cross as ways to make sure that prayer is always an integrated, body-soul experience.

Cultivate honest, but reverent, conversations about our bodies
The Holy Spirit speaks through the wisdom and counsel of our holy relationships. If there are themes in this book that speak to your heart, or challenge you to dig deeper, you can certainly do so on your own, but I would also encourage you to explore those ideas in community with other women. This doesn't mean that you can only talk about this with Catholic or even generally Christian women — so much can be gained through different perspectives! — but it does mean that you should seek out the

company of women who share your understanding of the dignity of the human body and are respectful of God's design of the human person.

If you'll allow your author to be so bold, I might directly suggest picking up this book and using it as a study or discussion guide. You could get a group together and form a book club, or share certain parts of this book with friends, sisters, and daughters whom you'd like to invite into this conversation together.

FINAL THOUGHTS

At a minimum, I pray that this text has helped you encounter the language of your body in a new or deeper way. Beyond that, it is my sincere prayer that we as the Church pay close attention to the signs of the times and encourage thoughtful reflection on new scientific information in light of the Gospel, so we never reduce the human person to a mere physical entity. In doing so, the Church will continue to be a beacon of truth, hope, and light for girls and women of all ages, who are searching for positive ways to integrate this unique aspect of feminine biology into their sense of self and their relationships. This is crucial for the Church in order to ensure that Catholics have an appreciation for the meaning of our bodies, which in turn fosters an appreciation for all of material creation, a deeper understanding of the sacraments, and a richer sense of God's unique design and plan for our vocation — whether that is to marriage, religious, or single life.

Whether our cycles are relatively easy, painfully challenging, or have completely gone missing, we need not be afraid to approach Christ. As we bring this book to a close, I'd like to offer one final reflection about a woman who did just that — so we return again to the woman who suffered from a hemorrhage.

In all three synoptic Gospels (Matthew, Mark, and Luke), we hear an account of a woman who had been bleeding for twelve years. It was understood that she had a ritual impurity, meaning that this bleeding was vaginal and that she was considered "unclean" for this entire time. While Luke, who was a physician, is typically associated with stories that include interesting medical descriptions, I actually prefer Mark's telling:

> And there was a woman who had had a flow of blood for twelve years, and who had suffered much under many physicians, and had spent all that she had, and was no better but rather grew worse. She had heard the reports about Jesus, and came up behind him in the crowd and touched his garment. For she said, "If I touch even his garments, I shall be made well." And immediately the hemorrhage ceased; and she felt in her body that she was healed of her disease. And Jesus, perceiving in himself that power had gone forth from him, immediately turned about in the crowd, and said, "Who touched my garments?" And his disciples said to him, "You see the crowd pressing around you, and yet you say, 'Who touched me?'" And he looked around to see who had done it. But the woman, knowing what had been done to her, came in fear and trembling and knelt down before him, and told him the whole truth. And he said to her, "Daughter, your faith has made you well; go in peace, and be healed of your disease." (Mk 5:25–34)

This woman spent all she had. She suffered under many physicians hoping for a cure, but in their hands her condition actually got worse. It would have been very simple for this woman to give up hope — according to Mosaic law, this woman had been ritually impure for more than a decade. Who knows what suffering she underwent in her relationships, in addition to the physical suffering of her body? But then she heard about Jesus, and despite the fact that she had not been permitted to even touch her husband for the whole period of her bleeding, she dared to reach out to Jesus with her "unclean" hands, and simply touch his garment.

I would like to put this woman forward as a powerful intercessor, not just for women who struggle with cycle-related health issues, but for any woman who is seeking to approach Jesus through coming to understand her menstrual cycle. This woman knew a fundamental truth that the apostles and presbyters needed a council to figure out: The incarnation of Jesus Christ has changed all of the rules. No longer must we make ourselves spiritually pure in order to approach God — through God taking on human form, it is now precisely our approach to him that makes us clean.

This lesson, gleaned from the gospel writers' accounts, provides plenty of food for thought; however, the tradition of our Church does not end the story of the hemorrhaging woman there. In both Eastern and Western traditions, this unnamed woman in the Gospel does not remain unnamed. Rather, the Church has traditionally given this woman the name *Veronica*.

Veronica is a name that means "true image." It's not found in the Bible, but the name might be familiar to those who have prayed the Stations of the Cross. In that particular devotion, the sixth station asks us to meditate upon the moment of Jesus' passion in which "Veronica wipes the face of Jesus." According to tradition, Jesus met a woman along the way to Calvary while he was carrying his cross. Moved with pity, the woman wiped the blood and sweat from Jesus' brow with her veil, upon which an imprint of his holy face miraculously appeared.

Could it be that the woman whose blood Jesus dried up with the touch of his cloth is the same woman who tradition says wiped the blood of Christ with her own cloth? We can ponder in our hearts what it might mean that the woman who suffered so greatly from blood was entrusted with safeguarding Christ's true image, written in blood.

Let us conclude this book in the same way we began, by approaching God in prayer:

In the name of the Father, and of the Son, and of the Holy Spirit.
Lord Jesus Christ, Divine Physician, and Son of Mary,
    teach us to see ourselves through the eyes of our Father.
Word of God, enlighten us to read the divine language written into our human nature,
    to receive the mystery of our feminine design as a gift,
    so we can make an authentic gift of self in whatever unique way you call us to holiness.
We especially ask for the intercession of our Blessed Mother in this task,
    along with Veronica and all the holy women who have walked before us in faith.
We thank you for sending your Spirit to be with us,
    and for the rich inheritance we have through the sacraments of the Church.
In Jesus' Holy Name we pray. Amen.

Explicit iste liber, scriptor sit crimine liber.

Acknowledgments

This book represents an attempt to weave together many threads of thought and experiences that I have collected over the years, so it's difficult for me to know where to start with acknowledgments because I have had so many fellow thread-collectors along the way!

It thus seems fitting to first mention my editor and now friend, Rebecca Martin, who was able to see the "heart need" for this book even when I couldn't yet articulate exactly what the project would look like. I am indebted both to her gentle encouragement and her astute editorial challenges, some of which I have saved in screenshots for times when I will need those reminders.

To Dr. Ross Angeli Bones-Castro, who has such a heart for this ministry and brings such a wealth of knowledge and joy. Special thanks goes to the very dear women in my life who previewed drafts of this particular book and offered their genuine feedback. To those sisters — Megan Haile, Danielle Killen, and Abby Walsh — I cannot thank you enough for the gift of your time and the sharing of your hearts that have so greatly shaped this text.

Gratitude is also due to Sister Laura, for impassioned conversations over cups of coffee that will stay with me for many years to come.

To Abby Jorgensen and Clare McCallan, my fellow word-crafters, cheerleaders, and support system through this whole process: Many, many thanks.

Going further back in time, I am deeply indebted to my undergraduate thesis advisor, Dr. Adrian J. Reimers, whose encouragement to expand John Paul II's *Theology of the Body* beyond conversations on marital intimacy has paved the way for so much prayer and thought in my life ever since.

To the men who so generously provided interviews and answered survey questions in order to craft our chapter on charting in the context of marriage: I hope you know what a gift it was to receive and be able to share your reflections. Thank you for your time and for speaking such beautiful, healing truths!

To all my BCC colleagues and friends, most notably Mikayla Dalton, whose invitation to become an instructor was obviously a turning point in my life. Her mentorship, friendship, and sisterhood in the Lay Dominicans are all great gifts.

To my clients, who have allowed me to walk with you for a short time in your own journeys of body literacy: Through your willingness to share your triumphs and challenges, I have gained such a deep appreciation for the kaleidoscope of experiences women and couples go through. Your witness is invaluable and greatly cherished. Thank you.

And finally, I must acknowledge those people whose presence is so inextricably woven into my own life that I cannot figure out how to articulate their impact. You alone walked with me and supported me through the whole writing process, which encompassed a period of time in our lives that required much fortitude and grace. To my parents and sisters, my wonderful in-laws: Thank you for the prayers and the encouragement.

To my husband and our children, who daily teach me to give and receive God's greatest gifts: I love you very much.

Christina Valenzuela
October 22, 2023
Feast of Pope St. John Paul II

Choosing an NFP Method

If you're looking to get started with cycle charting, you might be wondering how to choose which biomarkers to track and how to identify which method might be the best fit for you. There are certainly ways that you can pick up information about cycle tracking through various books, online resources, or even social media accounts. But if you want to maximize your benefit from using a method — whether that's specifically in the context of family planning or for health assessment — you will want to work with a trained instructor who can make sure you are properly understanding and applying the methodology.

This appendix is going to offer a little bit more detail about some of the common NFP methods that are available in the United States and then provide some commentary on what sorts of situations or preferences might lead someone to consider one method over another.

I will never take the position that there is a single "best method" over everything else. In my years of experience as an NFP instructor, I have observed:

1. It's quite possible for many different methods to work well for an individual or couple.
2. A method may be right for someone at one point in time, but not work well at another point in time.
3. Recommendations are never black and white: Some clients with very similar backgrounds will thrive in one method, while others will have difficulties, and it's not always apparent why.
4. It can be hard to know which biomarkers will work

well for you until you actually start trying to chart with them.

5. Some methods may feel really cumbersome to learn at first, but become much more comfortable over time as you gain experience, confidence, and more consistent habits.

For all of these reasons, I'd like you to give yourself permission to let go of the idea that you need to find the "perfect" method before committing to learning. That line of thinking can easily lead to decision paralysis. Instead, I much prefer to see women or couples do some very basic research and then make a good faith move to begin charting, assessing their comfort with a method as they learn more. This is also the reason I believe meeting with an instructor prior to booking a session is very important, because how well you communicate with and feel supported by your teacher can have a huge impact on your charting experience. When I have women or couples inquire about switching methods, I always am careful to see if I can identify whether their issues are actually with the method itself or with the instructor. I'd say in about thirty percent of the "switcher" inquiries I receive, it's the latter. If you haven't noticed yet, I'm very big on the importance of relationships.

So let's revisit the specific categories of methods that were briefly discussed in the chapter on charting, going a little more in-depth. Please note that websites may change and that this list is neither exhaustive nor representative of methods offered in general or USCCB approval for these methods. You can find a full list of USCCB-approved methods and providers at: usccb.org/topics /natural-family-planning/nfp-national-providers.

CERVICAL MUCUS METHODS

These methods observe and interpret cervical secretions to determine the timing of ovulation within a cycle.

Billings Ovulation Method
boma-usa.org

This method was pioneered in the 1950s by Australian husband and wife team Drs. John and Evelyn Billings, who created a system of identifying ovulation based on changes in cervical fluid patterns.[1] At the time, rhythm or calendar methods were the primary options available to couples for Natural Family Planning. Because those methods did not identify ovulation but simply worked off of statistical models of cycle fertility, the Billingses dubbed their new approach the "Ovulation Method." Eventually, as new approaches were developed, the method acquired their name and has since spread all over the world.

Billings offers an approach to charting that is customizable in terminology for the individual client, focusing on establishing a basic infertile pattern with cervical fluid observations. It utilizes sensation at the vulva and the appearance of secretions to distinguish different categories of fluid. Users who are uncomfortable with handling cervical secretions to determine texture and stretch may like this sort of approach.

Because it allows users to identify basic fertile and infertile patterns at various times throughout the cycle, Billings may be a very robust method for women or couples who experience irregular cycling patterns, either because they have a high degree of variability between the length of cycles, or because they routinely experience long cycles.

A side note: The cause for John and Evelyn's canonization is gaining popularity, and it is possible that they may become an officially recognized pair of married saints.

Creighton Model
creightonmodel.com

I find that Creighton is one of the more difficult methods to dive into when you're first trying to research NFP. What is CrMS? Na-

Pro? Is that different from FertilityCare? The terminology can seem confusing at first. So let's begin with a little bit of history on the method, just using the shorthand term "Creighton" for now.

At the most basic level, Creighton is a standardized system utilizing the Billings approach to classify cervical secretions. Whereas the Billings Ovulation Method can be flexible in terminology, Creighton is all about consistency and specifics, which has the benefit of being able to easily translate into consistent application of Creighton charts for healthcare. This approach was pioneered in the late 1970s by Dr. Thomas Hilgers and continues with research, primarily through the Saint Paul VI Institute, to this day. This is partly why there are different terms that can apply to this method. The actual method of observation and charting is called the Creighton Model Fertility*Care* System, or CrMS. The health science that utilizes this system for diagnostics and treatment is called NaProTECHNOLOGY, or Natural Procreative Technology. A Fertility*Care* Practitioner (FCP) is a person who teaches you how to chart with CrMS.

Who might this system work well for? I find that women who are very detail-oriented and like to get a lot of information from a single fertility sign tend to do well with this method long term. There are a lot of medical situations in which charting with Creighton will be helpful, and many NaPro providers will exclusively work with CrMS charts. So even if Creighton isn't necessarily your method of choice for the long haul, some women and couples do find it to be incredibly helpful for assisting with particular health concerns. Examples of those situations could be endometriosis investigation and treatment, infertility, hormonal imbalances, and ovarian cysts.

Two-Day Method
irh.org/twoday-method
This method was developed by the Institute for Reproductive Health at Georgetown University as a simple way to monitor cervical secretions. Checks are done at least twice a day to determine

the presence of cervical fluid. If today and yesterday were both dry, then today is considered an infertile day. The benefit of this approach is that it can be learned very quickly, in a single instructional session with a provider. It also requires no additional technology, no special equipment (even a chart would be optional), and can be taught even in populations with lower education and literacy rates.

SYMPTO-THERMAL METHODS

These methods utilize cervical fluid and basal body temperature to determine the timing of ovulation within a cycle. In speaking with several instructors across different methods, I find that the biggest differences between these organizations are less about their specific charting protocols — which look very similar and yield similar interpretive patterns of fertility/infertility — and are more about their teaching philosophies and modalities. What follows are quick summaries of each:

Couple to Couple League
ccli.org

This method was developed by John and Sheila Kippley in the late 1970s, with help from Dr. Konald Prem. One of the unique aspects of this method is found within the name: "Couple." Instruction in the method is delivered by a trained volunteer couple, rather than an individual, in response to the call issued in *Humanae Vitae*:

> Among the fruits that ripen if the law of God be resolutely obeyed, the most precious is certainly this, that married couples themselves will often desire to communicate their own experience to others. Thus it comes about that in the fullness of the lay vocation will be included a novel and outstanding form of the apostolate by which, like ministering to like, married couples themselves by

the leadership they offer will become apostles to other married couples. (26)

Thus CCL is a highly recommended method for couples who specifically want to receive education and support from another couple, keeping in mind that learning together as a couple is the ideal, but is not strictly required. This program also has an emphasis on teaching the benefits of breastfeeding.

SymptoPro
symptopro.org

This method was originally developed and delivered under the name Northwest Family Services, with direct support from researcher Dr. Josef Roetzer. Unlike other organizations which primarily focus on NFP, Northwest Family Services is a larger organization that seeks to bring stability to families and promote the well-being of children by linking health to meaningful social and support services. So, you could perhaps say that SymptoPro is part of NWFS's vision of family "health" and social justice, which wouldn't necessarily impact the experience of utilizing the method, but contextualizes it in a broader community vision.

NFP International
nfpandmore.org

This is the second NFP organization that claims John and Sheila Kippley as founders. Founded in 2004 after the Kippleys left CCL, NFP International is rooted in a unique educational philosophy that emphasizes what the Kippleys call a "triple-strand approach" to NFP: instruction on ecological breastfeeding, the foundations of covenant theology, and systematic family planning that allows couples freedom of choice with minimum abstinence.

HORMONAL METHODS

This category of method originally included the combination of cervical fluid and urinary hormone testing, garnering the label "symptohormonal." However, the inclusion of basal body temperature and the increasing popularity of exclusive hormone testing suggest that a better categorical move would be to drop the "sympto" element in the terminology.

Marquette Model
marquette.edu/nursing/natural-family-planning-model.php

The Marquette Model was a completely innovative approach to fertility charting, pioneered in the early 2000s by lead researcher Dr. Richard Fehring at Marquette University's Institute for Natural Family Planning at the College of Nursing. This novel approach sought to utilize readily available technologies of hormone monitoring to help couples accurately identify their fertile window for family planning. They eventually created a system that incorporated fluid and temperature protocols around the Clearblue® Fertility Monitor, which measures both estradiol and LH. Because of these origins, the Marquette Model continues to be both innovative and research-driven. Its nursing school ties are also reflected in the method's requirement for instructors to have professional healthcare credentials (a minimum of a BSN).

Therefore, Marquette might be your preferred method if you want to work with hormonal testing and have a strong desire to receive instruction from a healthcare professional. If you have a specific medical condition that you need help navigating with charting, you can also seek out an instructor who has specifically taken the Medical Applications course.

Boston Cross Check
bostoncrosscheck.com

This is the method that I am certified to teach, so it holds a special place in my heart. But I still will insist that this is not necessarily the best method for everyone! The origins of Boston Cross Check go back to the 1970s, when this local sympto-thermal method was part of the New England NFP Association. It was renamed in 2005 and remained an in-house method for the Archdiocese of Boston for many years. As an organization, BCC is probably the smallest of the methods listed here, with fewer than two dozen certified instructors worldwide. But because it's the method I know most about, it's going to be included here! BCC is a slightly more conservative method in some respects, meaning it will sometimes calculate a larger fertile window than other methods (and therefore mean a little more abstinence). Protocols are designed for maximum flexibility: Users learn a standard toolkit of observations with fluid, temps, and how to work with the Clearblue® Fertility Monitor, but are not required to chart all signs. Additional options with LH testing or PdG testing are also approved. This approach tends to be preferred by couples who want the additional peace of mind offered by calculating a longer fertile window, or who prefer to collect a lot of different data points.

FEMM Health
femmhealth.org
In some ways, this method is perhaps the most philosophically distinct within our list here. Rather than originally being developed around family planning and fertility, FEMM was created to teach cycle charting in the context of holistic women's health and medical management. By no means is this application unique to FEMM (we have already seen that Creighton and Marquette include some robust support in the sphere of healthcare), but it does mean that the method has been crafted in such a way that it might appeal to a broader audience at the outset. I include FEMM in the hormonal method category because it uses cervical mucus and LH testing, although it could also be considered an ovulation

method with optional hormonal monitoring.

THINGS TO CONSIDER

Various factors may lead someone to choose one method over another. For many of us, accessibility and familiarity will be the leading deciding factor. If you happen to know an instructor personally, or have a particular method promoted in your local parish, it may make sense to just go with what is available. However, many instructors will teach remotely or will have self-paced learning options, so it's not necessarily the case that a local instructor is any more or less accessible than one who lives many time zones away.

There are a few things to consider about utilizing particular biomarkers — with the caveat that there could be exceptions, and it's always worth asking a potential instructor specifically about how his or her method would approach these situations.

It could be difficult to get cervical fluid readings if you:

- have persistent yeast infections or cervical ectropion, which obscures fluid signs
- have constant fluid signs and are not confident finding an infertile pattern
- have frequent bleeding/spotting episodes throughout the cycle that obscure fluid
- are uncomfortable observing secretions for any reason
- are taking medications that impact cervical fluid production or presentation
- find it difficult to get in the habit of making regular checks

It could be difficult to get reliable basal body temps if you:

- have an irregular sleep schedule

- frequently travel across time zones
- work changing shifts throughout the month
- take certain steroids
- use progesterone treatment (although in some cases you can wait to begin progesterone supplementation until you have verified a temp shift)
- experience high levels of stress or other factors that disturb your sleep
- experience elevated temperatures after consuming alcohol

Note that some of these scenarios can be worked around by utilizing a wearable thermometer, instead of doing traditional oral temping.

It could be difficult to monitor hormones if you:

- are frequently dehydrated
- are unable to test consistently during the required days
- regularly take antibiotics such as tetracycline, which can interfere with LH readings
- have persistently high levels of LH due to PCOS or other conditions
- regularly have cycles longer than forty days

These are just a very few situations that are related to specific biomarkers. Additionally, consider your personality and preferences when choosing a method.

Do you prefer to work with a lot of data, or a little bit of data? If you like to keep things simple, then a single-indicator approach such as Billings or even the monitor-only protocols with Marquette might be your choice. But if you like to have a lot of data, you can think about whether you'd like a lot of detail about a single sign (perhaps Creighton for you) or data points about multiple different signs (BCC or Marquette with all the options).

Do you typically "trust" technology? I have a lot of clients who think they want a lot of different data points, but when it comes down to the application, they tell me they don't actually trust a monitor or a wearable thermometer that uses an algorithm. They worry that something has gone wrong with the technology, so they end up being anxious with the data, rather than confident. In this case, a cervical mucus method or a sympto-thermal method with a simple oral BBT might be a more comfortable approach.

Are you very consistent, or do you need shortcuts? Every method requires the formation of consistent habits to ensure that you are getting the data that you need. But some methods need less data than others. If you are someone who works better with a consistent routine every day, then go all-in with checking cervical fluid and/or temping every day. But if you do better with shorter bursts of consistency, then maybe you want to utilize hormone testing with or without a cross-check that you are able to drop after confirming ovulation.

What's your learning style? Not all methods offer self-paced video courses. Some methods are primarily group classes, while others are more one-on-one. Be sure the method you are considering can be delivered in a way that is comfortable and most effective for you.

INSTRUCTOR DIRECTORIES

As of publication, the following general (not method-specific) directories are available to assist women and couples in finding an instructor. Please note that Catholics will want to filter through any directory options, to ensure that instructors are teaching methods and utilizing protocols that are consonant with Church teaching (i.e., not recommending barriers or other backup options).

- FACTS About Fertility: factsaboutfertility.org/physician -clinician-educator-directory/
- Fertility Science Institute Directory: fertilityscienceinstitute .org/directory/
- My Catholic Doctor: mycatholicdoctor.com/fertility -educators/
- One More Soul Directory: onemoresoul.com/nfp-directory
- Read Your Body Educators Directory: readyourbody.com /educators-directory/

NOTES

Chapter 1

1. Jane Knight, *The Complete Guide to Fertility Awareness* (New York: Routledge, 2017), 14–26.

2. "Menstruation: A Nonadaptive Consequence of Uterine Evolution," *The Quarterly Review of Biology* 73, no. 2 (June 1998): 163-173, https://pubmed.ncbi.nlm.nih.gov/9618925/.

3. If you'd like a less-folksy version, my pal Thomas Aquinas has a wonderful exploration of original sin and the rupture of original justice in the *Summa Theologiae*, First Part of the Second Part, Question 85.

4. Edith Stein, *The Collected Works of Edith Stein*, Vol II: Essays on Women, ed. L. Gelber, trans. F. Oben, Ph.D. (Washington, DC: ICS Publications, 2017), 63.

5. *Apostolic Constitutions*, trans. James Donaldson, from *Ante-Nicene Fathers*, vol. 7., ed. Alexander Roberts, James Donaldson, and A. Cleveland Coxe (Buffalo, NY: Christian Literature Publishing Co., 1886). Revised and edited for New Advent by Kevin Knight, http://www.newadvent.org/fathers/0715.htm, Book VI, XXIII.

6. Hildegard von Bingen, *On Natural Philosophy and Medicine: Selections from Cause et Cure,* trans. Margret Berger (Cambridge: D. S. Brewer, 1999), 90.

7. Ambrose of Milan, *Hexameron, Paradise, and Cain and Abel*, trans. John J. Savage (New York: Fathers of the Church, Inc., 1961), 434.

Chapter 2

1. "Menstruation in Girls and Adolescents: Using the Menstrual Cycle as a Vital Sign," Committee Opinion no. 651, American College of Obstetricians and Gynecologists, Obstetrics & Gynecology 126 (2015): 143–146.

Chapter 3

1. *The Baltimore Catechism,* rev. ed 1941, The Mary Foundation,

https://www.catholicity.com/baltimore-catechism/.

2. Barbara Newman, "Commentary on the Johannine Prologue: Hildegard of Bingen," *Theology Today* 60, Part 1, Vision 4, Chapter 105 (2003): 16–33.

3. *On the Origin of Humanity*, Discourse 1: pp 31-32

4. R. Shane Tubbs et al., *History of Anatomy: An International Perspective* (Hoboken, NJ: Wiley Blackwell, 2019), 154.

5. Edith Stein, *The Collected Works of Edith Stein, Vol II: Essays on Women*, ed. L. Gelber, trans. F. Oben, Ph.D. (Washington, DC: ICS Publications, 2017), 197.

Chapter 4

1. *The Summa Theologiæ of St. Thomas Aquinas,* Second and Revised Edition, trans. Fathers of the English Dominican Province, https://www.newadvent.org/summa/2001.html.

2. As can sometimes happen with induced amenorrhea, where our bodies lack sufficient fuel, enter "starvation mode," and cease with our cycles until a healthier state is restored.

Chapter 5

1. *Catechism of the Catholic Church*, 2558.

2. "Constitution on the Sacred Liturgy," *The Liturgy Documents: A Parish Resource*, ed. David Lysik, (Chicago: Liturgy Training Publications, 2004), 5.

3. "Praying with Body, Mind, and Voice," United States Conference of Catholic Bishops, 2010, https://www.usccb.org/prayer-and-worship/the-mass/upload/praying-with-body-mind-and-voice.pdf.

4. Martin Connell, *Eternity Today: On the Liturgical Year,* vol. 1 (New York: The Continuum International Publishing Group, 2006), 5.

5. Thomas Aquinas, *Commentary on the Gospel of John: Chapters 9–21*, trans. Fabian Larcher (Lander, WY: The Aquinas Institute for the Study of Sacred Doctrine, 2013), 450.

Chapter 6

1. G. K. Chesterton, *Orthodoxy* (San Francisco: Ignatius Press, 1995), 66.

2. Thomas Aquinas, "Adoro te Devote/Godhead Here in Hiding," trans. Gerard Manley Hopkins, Hymnary.org, 2023, https://hymnary.org/text/godhead_here_in_hiding.

3. Julian of Norwich. *Revelations of Divine Love* (Grand Rapids, MI: Christian Classics Ethereal Library, 2002), www.ccel.org/julian/revelations/html.

4. Caryll Houselander, *The Dry Wood* (Providence, RI: Cluny Media, 2021), 152.

Chapter 7

1. The etymology of the term is admittedly uncertain: Possibly it came from an older German phrase *Gottes Freitag,* meaning "God's Friday," or it may also reflect interchangeable usage between the words "good" and "holy." Whatever the origin, we can take the resulting name as an opportunity for theological reflection on goodness and fittingness.

2. Chaya Raichik, *Mikvah Stories: A Collection of True Stories of Women Overcoming Today's Challenges* (New Brunswick, NJ: Targum Publishing, 2022), 13. Note: *Hashem* is a Jewish placeholder term meaning "The Name" and is used to refer to God where we might instead place the Tetragrammaton YHWH, as given in Exodus 3.

3. Bonni Goldberg, *Reclaiming Mikvah: Embracing Jewish Water Ritual* (Portland, OR: Vizye Publications, 2017), 9–10.

4. This note is going to be a side note for anyone who is wondering about whether the Church has ever prohibited women from worship (specifically, from receiving the Eucharist) while experiencing menstruation. The complicated answer is primarily no, but kind of yes? Evidence for excluding menstruating women is found in the *Corpus Juris Canonici,* which might be considered a sort of precursor to the Code of Canon Law of 1917. Within that document exist collections of writings that range

greatly in their actual juridical value. In other words, some parts are very authoritative and binding, and others not so much. Because we also have evidence from the Apostolic Constitutions, Gregory the Great, and others that directly contradicts the proscriptions in the *Corpus Juris* (that is, they expressly do NOT prohibit women from receiving the Eucharist while menstruating), then it is reasonable to surmise that even if exclusion happened in particular times and places, it was never a highly authoritative or universal practice of the Church. For more information see:

- Alphonse Van Hove, "Corpus Juris Canonici," *The Catholic Encyclopedia,* vol. 4 (New York: Robert Appleton Co., 1908), http://www.newadvent.org/cathen/04391a.htm.
- *The Apostolic Constitutions,* Vol. 7, trans. James Donaldson, eds. Alexander Roberts, James Donaldson, and A. Cleveland Coxe, from Ante-Nicene Fathers (Buffalo, NY: Christian Literature Publishing Co., 1886), revised and edited for New Advent by Kevin Knight, http://www.newadvent.org/fathers/0715.htm.
- Gregory the Great, *Registrum Epistolarum,* Second Series, vol. 13, trans. James Barmby, ed. Philip Schaff and Henry Wace, from Nicene and Post-Nicene Fathers (Buffalo, NY: Christian Literature Publishing Co., 1898), revised and edited for New Advent by Kevin Knight. http://www.newadvent.org/fathers/360211064.htm.

5. Melito of Sardis, "Easter Homily," *The Liturgy of the Hours: Vol. II* (New York: Catholic Book Publishing Corp., 1976), 459.

6. "Office of Readings for Good Friday," *The Liturgy of the Hours: Book II: Lenten Season, Easter Season* (New York: Catholic Publishing Group, 1976).

7. See, for reference, the work of Beth Williamson, "The Virgin Lactans as Second Eve: Image of the 'Salvatrix,'" *Studies in Iconography,* vol. 19 (1998): 105–38, http://www.jstor.org/stable/23923610.

8. Ernest Brehaut, *An Encyclopedist of the Dark Ages: Isidore of Seville* (New York: Columbia University Press, 1912).

9. Saint Bonaventure, *The Life of Saint Francis,* trans. and ed. Ewert Cousins (Mahwah, NJ: Paulist Press, 1976), 306.

10. See Richard A. Lord, "A Note On Stigmata," *American Imago* 14, no. 3 (1957): 299–302, http://www.jstor.org/stable/26301636.

11. See Augustin Poulain, "Mystical Stigmata," *The Catholic Encyclopedia*, vol. 14 (New York: Robert Appleton Company, 1912), http://www.newadvent.org/cathen/14294b.htm.

12. Caroline Walker Bynum, *Holy Feast and Holy Fast: The Religious Significance of Food to Medieval Women* (Berkeley: University of California Press, 1987), 274.

13. Pope St. John Paul II, "Homily: Beatification of Six Servants of God," April 25, 2004, vatican.va.

Chapter 8

1. See St. Paul's explanation in Romans 5 and 1 Corinthians 15.

2. Irenaeus, *Against Heresies,* trans. A. Roberts and W. Rambaut, from *Ante-Nicene Fathers*, vol. 1, ed. Alexander Roberts, James Donaldson, and A. Cleveland Coxe (Buffalo, NY: Christian Literature Publishing Co., 1885.) Revised and edited for New Advent by Kevin Knight, www.newadvent.org/fathers/0103322.htm.

3. Thomas Aquinas, Suppl. Q 81 Art 4, sed contra

4. Hildegard von Bingen, *Scivias: Book One,* trans. Mother Columba Hart and Jane Bishop (New York: Paulist Press, 1990), 87.

5. "Ancient Homily on Holy Saturday," *The Liturgy of the Hours: Book II* (New York: Catholic Book Publishing Corp.,1976).

6. Gregory of Nazianzus, *Letter to Cledonius the Priest Against Apollinarius,* trans. C. G. Browne and J. E. Swallow. From *Nicene and Post-Nicene Fathers,* Second Series, vol. 7, ed. P. Schaff and H. Wace. (Buffalo, NY: Christian Literature Publishing Co., 1894). Revised and edited for New Advent by Kevin Knight, http://www.newadvent.org/fathers/3103a.htm.

7. Felix Just, "Basic Texts for the Roman Catholic Eucharist," Eucharistic Prayers I–IV, from the 3rd ed. of the *Roman Missal,* English Translation, 2011, 18 Jan 2022. www.catholic-resources.org. 9 Mar 2023.

8. "I adore you devoutly, O hidden God." From the text of the hymn by the same name, composed for the feast of Corpus Christi.

9. Louis de Montfort, *True Devotion to Mary with Preparation for Total Consecration* (Charlotte: TAN Books, 2010), 1.

10. Teresa of Avila, *The Interior Castle: Study Edition,* 2nd ed., trans. K. Kavanaugh (Washington, DC: ICS Publications, 2020), 6.4.16.

11. Fulton J. Sheen, *The World's First Love: Mary the Mother of God,* 2nd ed. (San Francisco: Ignatius Press, 2010), 51.

12. I am working from memory with these quotations, since I did not record these reflections! In some cases, I expect I am conflating a couple of different women's thoughts. And I know that I have not managed to capture all the beautiful things that have been shared.

13. John of Damascus, *Three Treatises on the Divine Images,* trans. Louth (Crestwood: St. Vladimir's Seminary Press, 2003), 46.

Chapter 9

1. It is important to note that some types of hormonal contraceptives are less reliable in this particular function, and will then have a "back up" effect of preventing implantation after conception has occurred. This is more common for the progesterone-only (non-combination) formulations. For more information, please visit: https:/www.ncbcenter.org/resources-and-statements-cms/summary-abortion-contraception-and-responsible-parenthood-february-2013.

2. "How Paragard Works." October 2022. https://www.paragard.com/how-paragard-works/

Chapter 10

1. Francis de Sales. *Introduction to the Devout Life,* Catholic Spiritual Direction, Part II, Chapter IX, 2017, https://catholicspiritualdirection.org/devoutlife.pdf.

Chapter 11

1. For this articulation, I am indebted to the work of Christopher K. Gross, Ph.D., who wrote a dissertation entitled *Men and Women Becoming Virtuous: An Examination of Aquinas's Theory of Virtue in Light of a Contemporary Account of Sexual Difference*, published by Catholic University of America in 2013.

2. The word *askesis* in Greek means "exercise," like what an athlete would do to train for a marathon. It was also applied to the moral life, to indicate the moral "exercise" of virtue-building, and was later taken up in a particular way by the Christian Desert Fathers, who became knowns as "ascetics," or the "athletes" who train in a particular way to win the imperishable crown (cf. 1 Cor9:24–27).

3. Dan Burke, *Spiritual Warfare and the Discernment of Spirits* (Manchester: Sophia Institute Press, 2019), 90.

Chapter 12

1. For a summary of estrogen and progesterone effects on the brain, see Kaitlyn McOsker, "Hormonal Balance and the Female Brain: A Review," FACTS, May 10 2021, https://www.factsaboutfertility.org/hormonal-balance-and-the-female-brain-a-review/.

2. There is a technical, but nonstandard, medical usage of this term that is not consistent with popular usage. I tend to avoid use of the term but acknowledge its meaning when used colloquially in this way.

3. See A. D. Domar, P. C. Zuttermeister, and R. Friedman, "The Psychological Impact of Infertility: A Comparison with Patients with Other Medical Conditions," *Journal of Psychosomatic Obstetrics and Gynaecology*, 1993, 14 Suppl: 45–52, PMID: 8142988.

4. Thomas Aquinas, *Summa Contra Gentiles*, trans. Rickaby, public domain. Electronic version copyright *The Catholic Primer*, Book IV, LV, 17, https://www.catholicprimer.org/.

Chapter 13

1. Hanna Klaus, Nora Dennehy, and Jean Turnbull, "Undergirding

Abstinence Within a Sexuality Education Program," October 21, 2001, www.lifeissues.net/writers/kla/kla_02abstinenceedu1.html.

2. As a side note, it's worth mentioning that while writing this book, countries in Europe have begun to offer menstrual leave legislation, adding to a handful of similar policies around the world. Debate continues to ensue about whether these policies help women or harm them by playing into misguided ideas about biological determinism, and increasing the number of biology-based reasons why an employer would want to discriminate against women in hiring practices. I acknowledge the difficulties of these legal questions, while maintaining that at the interpersonal level, there is only good to be gained by accepting one another for the way God has designed us to work.

3. See J. F. Fraumeni Jr., J. W. Lloyd, E. M. Smith, and J. K. Wagoner, "Cancer Mortality Among Nuns: Role of Marital Status in Etiology of Neoplastic Disease in Women," *Journal of the National Cancer Institute* 42, 3 (March 1969): 455–468, PMID: 5777491.

Chapter 14

1. See, for example, Richard J. Fehring and Michael D. Manhart, "Natural Family Planning and Marital Chastity: The Effects of Periodic Abstinence on Marital Relationships," *The Linacre Quarterly* 88, 1 (2021): 42–55, doi:10.1177/0024363920930875.

Chapter 15

1. Lara Briden, *The Hormone Repair Manual: Every Woman's Guide to Healthy Hormones after 40* (Middletown: Greenpeak Publishing, 2021), 28.

2. Ibid., 29.

3. Chesterton, *Orthodoxy*, 66.

4. Simon Tugwell, *The Beatitudes: Soundings in Christian Tradition* (Springfield: Templegate Publishers, 1980), 6–7.

5. See, for example, D Frank and T Williams, "Attitudes about Menstruation among Fifth-, Sixth-, and Seventh-grade Pre- and

Post-Menarcheal Girls," *The Journal of School Nursing* 15 (1999): 25–31.

    6. CCC 916.

    7. For examples of this, see M. L. Marván and M. Molina-Abolnik, "Mexican Adolescents' Experience of Menarche and Attitudes Toward Menstruation: Role of Communication Between Mothers and Daughters," *Journal of Pediatric and Adolescent Gynecology* 25, 6 (December 2012): 358–363, doi: 10.1016/j.jpag.2012.05.003. Epub 2012 Sep 11. PMID: 22975203. D Frank and T Williams, "Attitudes about Menstruation among Fifth-, Sixth-, and Seventh-grade Pre- and Post-Menarcheal Girls," *The Journal of School Nursing* 15 (1999): 25–31. doi: 10.1177/105984059901500405. PMID: 10818878.

    8. Jess Connolly, *Breaking Free from Body Shame: Dare to Reclaim What God Has Named Good* (Grand Rapids, MI: Zondervan Books, 2021), 28.

    9. Pontifical Council for the Family, "The Truth and Meaning of Human Sexuality: Guidelines for Education Within the Family," December 8, 1995, vatican.va.

    10. Ibid.

    11. "Biblia Sacra Vulgata," Bible Gateway, 2023, biblegateway.com.

Conclusion

    1. Hildegard von Bingen, *Causae et Curae,* trans. Margret Berger (Rochester, NY: D.S. Brewer, 1999), 124.

Appendix

    1. I will utilize the term cervical "fluid" because this is the demonstrated preference that my clients like, and what I am most comfortable using. However, the term most commonly used by other NFP methods is cervical "mucus," which is helpful because it reinforces the connection for charters that our cervical secretions can be impacted any time our general mucus patterns are affected in the body, as in times of illness or under the

effects of certain medications. Please keep in mind that the terms "cervical fluid" and "cervical mucus" are interchangeable here, and if you are searching online you may want to use the term "mucus" in order to yield more complete search results.

About the Author

Christina Valenzuela is the owner and creative director of Pearl & Thistle, LLC, where she offers a unique blend of theology and science to bring better body literacy to Catholic families and parishes. She has been a certified instructor in the Boston Cross Check™ method of Natural Family Planning since 2013, and her signature "Cycle Prep: First Period Course" was a 2021 OSV Innovation Challenge finalist. She holds an undergraduate degree in philosophy and theology from the University of Notre Dame as well as a master's in theological studies from Harvard Divinity School. Christina is a life-professed member of the Lay Fraternities of Saint Dominic and resides with her husband and children outside of Boston. You can learn more about her work at pearlandthistle.com.